2d

P9-DCU-244

YOGA
AND HEALTH

YOGA
AND HEALTH

By Selvarajan Yesudian
and Elisabeth Haich

Translated by John P. Robertson

Harper & Brothers
Publishers . New York

YOGA AND HEALTH

Copyright, 1953, by Harper & Brothers

Printed in the United States of America

All rights in this book are reserved.
No part of the book may be used or reproduced
in any manner whatsoever without written per-
mission except in the case of brief quotations
embodied in critical articles and reviews. For
information address Harper & Brothers
49 East 33rd Street, New York 16, N. Y.

Library of Congress catalog card number: 54-6039

Foreword
BY THE AUTHOR

PROMPTED by an inner urge which I could not disobey, I left India and came to Europe. I acted as a tool in the hands of destiny and, like a vessel into which a liquid is poured, I accepted everything it gave me. I found no rest until I had received the answer to my greatest, my only question—Man; for now I know:

> Man, thou art thy secret alone!
> Who can ope thy gates but thee?
> And none to enter in but thee!

Man is a mysterious marvel, moving between the two death-bringing factors of time and space. The fact that his days are numbered requires him to awaken out of his dreamy slumbers and recognise the power of his being and the limitlessness of his SELF. In his heart man feels the dawning of exalted happiness in its golden glory and immortal magnificence, and he awakens to the realization that his true nature is nothing but bliss.

Following this inner voice, I decided to write down all I had seen and learned, in the hope that my experiences might serve as a useful guide for others engaged in the same search.

I have no wish to propagate Orientalism or a cult of any kind. True and enduring happiness, however, can only be attained in a healthy frame. For this reason I am mentioning some long-established rules and precepts which can be useful for achieving success. They have been compiled in such a way as to correspond to the requirements of those Occidentals who are willing to sacrifice a blind and purposeless activity to the extent of devoting a few minutes daily to self-development.

The struggle for health is hard, and the victor must conquer both body and soul. Secrets are waiting to be revealed when, like a bud unfolding into a blossom, this mystery of man is solved and the majesty of man's true being is made manifest. But this requires time and patient work. Like a gardener, one can make his way towards successful realization only if body and soul are brought to obey, in unison, the commands of the immortal Overself dwelling within. As the brain develops, like the unfolding of the delicate petals of a flower, and as the body grows towards physical perfection, the Overself expresses itself as perfect health, perception, and knowledge. Be conscious as a whole and you will reach this goal.

Our world today needs health more than anything that wealth has to offer. To prevent the causes of sickness and suffering is just as sacred a task as to bring about the healing for which millions are so desperately yearning. Begin, therefore, by refusing to tolerate any negative influences—either mental or physical; for disease is a lack of positive life force, a void in the constitution which ends in the collapse of the system. The ancient science of Yoga is as perfect as it is exact, in that it points out those wise and sensible steps that must be taken in order to achieve physical and mental perfection.

My work has been more than abundantly seconded and advanced through the assistance of Elisabeth Haich who is not only my colleague in our Yoga School, but has also helped me to interpret the exact requirements of the Occident. We have written this book together, based upon the experiences of long hard years of work and a rich harvest of encouraging results. These pages have been written for those who are unable to visit a Yoga school or an 'ashram' and who do not have the good luck to be able to find a personal guide. We earnestly hope that this book will enable the diligent seeker to perform the exercises and travel upon the conscious path of Hatha Yoga.

> To see, open then thine eyes,
> And behold below the veil of
> blindness, that mortal flesh
> covereth . . . MAN the DIVINE.

SELVARAJAN YESUDIAN

Contents

Illustrations

PART 1

I

_ _ _ _ _

True Story of a Sick Boy

ONCE there lived in sunny India, in the city of Madras, a thin
and sickly little boy. By his fifteenth birthday he had had almost
every major disease—scarlet fever, dysentery, typhus, cholera,
and the other contagious diseases so common in the tropics.
It was little short of a miracle that he was still alive. He sur-
vived indeed, but in what a deplorable condition! He was only
skin and bones. His little face was peaked, his eyes hollowed
and sunken, his chest narrow and flat. And yet this little boy
never was in want. On the contrary, his father was a famous
and wealthy physician to whom the sick flocked in a steady
stream. His mother was the sweetest, gentlest mother in the
world. Nevertheless this house in Madras, with its big shady
courtyard, knew no happiness. Constant worry and affliction
were the lot of its inhabitants; for the closely guarded
and coddled little child looked more like a shadow than a
boy.

His father tried every means known to medicine. But he
barely succeeded in keeping his son alive.

One day the boy was sent to school. Now he was no longer
obliged to lie down hour after hour, as in the past. From
this moment on he was able to live like the other little boys of
his age. Naturally he was exempted from gymnastics, and at
home he was shielded, as in the past, from every breath of air.
When he was fourteen, he caught pneumonia, but again, as if
by a miracle, he managed to pull through. The endless care and
trouble began anew. Half a year later he was fairly well again,
but took cold at the merest draught. Words can hardly express
how much this poor little boy envied his happy school com-

panions with their rugged health. During the gym classes in the English high school he withdrew into a corner of the courtyard where with heavy heart and yearning glances, he watched the agile movements of the other boys. When the class was over, he stayed on in the court and, as soon as he felt himself unobserved, ran and jumped around, swinging his arms about, just as he had seen the others do. At fifteen he felt better. The colds did not come so often now; but the irregular and surreptitiously practised gymnastic exercises gave him headaches and palpitations of the heart.

Despite the frailty of his body, his spirit of initiative was unbroken. Often he ran away, wandering through field and forest in search of Yogi settlements, so-called ashrams, in the far-off hills. But his efforts were fruitless, and so he contented himself with gazing at the itinerant fakirs who demonstrated their prowess beside the road. While he thought little of these fakirs, he was full of admiration for the real Yogis. Thanks to an inborn instinct, he was drawn towards the mystic science of ancient India. He read every book he could find on the subject in his father's library. He knew and admired the theory of the spiritual sciences: the teachings of Raja Yoga, Jnana Yoga and Karma Yoga which open up joyous spiritual heights and confer contentment, faith, and strength of soul upon their disciples. He also found numerous books on Hatha Yoga which contained the secret rules, simple though many milleniums old, for attaining physical well-being, strength, and health. The enthusiasm of a child with such a weak constitution can easily be imagined. Almost in one fell swoop, from early afternoon until night and right on again until dawn—he devoured the contents of the newly discovered books. He shouted for joy as he read about 'asanas,' the Yoga postures, and breathing exercises which bring strength and health. On the spot, he sat up in bed, crossing his legs after the fashion described in the first exercise. Then, one after another, he tried to imitate all the important postures; with the result that he nearly dislocated his legs. Meanwhile, having read that deep breathing is of particular importance in human life, he tried the pranayama breathing exercises. Filling up his weak lungs, he held his breath until he almost burst. Then he stood on his head and twisted

16

his arms and legs about until, to cap the climax, he tumbled out of bed, bumped his head a resounding whack, and roused the whole household from a sound sleep. After long hours of such over-exertion, his gasping lungs were ready to burst. The next day found him weak and miserable, aching in every joint. After a week's efforts he put the books aside, crying bitter tears. The thought that even this last chance to achieve physical strength was cut off made him disconsolate. He gave up hope, believing that he would never be healthy, never be able to romp and wrestle with his playmates . . . never be able to enjoy the happiness that comes with sturdy, carefree youth.

From then on he became uncommunicative. He despised the body and interested himself only in things of the spirit. But just learning lessons and reading a great deal failed to satisfy him. More and more his attention was drawn to problems too serious and too deep for his age.

On a sultry autumn evening he ran away again. In a mango grove a few miles from the city, he found—at last!—the long-sought Hatha Yogi master!

The Yogi was surrounded by a group of young people who were listening to his teaching. During the lesson the young boy remained in hiding, watching the group from a distance. He saw that the young men had beautiful bodies with splendid muscles and that they were performing strange exercises. He also noticed that they were glowing with health. When the group broke up, the youngster approached the master and asked him humbly to accept him as a pupil.

Two months later the Madras doctor hardly recognised his son. Now the boy walked straight as an arrow. His chest had deepened. His shoulders were growing broader every day. At the end of a year his chest had expanded four inches. His arms and legs had almost doubled in size. From then on he was never sick again. At school, without ever having taken part in the English gymnastic lessons, he had become the most dex-terous—over night!

When he was twenty, after the death of his father, he travelled again to a distant city to visit his master to whom, after God and his parents, he owed health, strength, and even life itself. He told his master that he had felt an inner call to undertake a

17

long journey to Europe. After a touching farewell, his master said:

"Go, my boy, and get acquainted with the West. Compare the people of the West with those of the East—the way of the Occident with that of the Orient—and see where the two paths meet. Learn from the people of the Occident the things in which they are ahead of us, and make known to them the things in which the Orient has already reached the goal. Go and work in your way to help bring these two paths together. But in the West you will realize that the science of Hatha Yoga is not only the way to health, but also the world's only physical culture method based on the close union between body and soul. Although it is a science for building up the *body*, it is nevertheless based on *mental* and *spiritual* forces."

The boy looked with shining eyes at his master, folded his hands and bowed.—"Master, I knew this a long time ago when I was endeavouring to build up my body. When I directed my attention to the different parts of my body . . . my muscles and nerve centres, I noticed that hitherto unknown spiritual powers developed within me. To the extent that I became master of my body, my will power increased. You brought me back to life; you took a sickly, emaciated little boy and turned him into an athlete. You took me out of physical ruin and led me back to myself! I promise you. . . ."

"Promise nothing, my boy! . . . The West is in a turmoil and seems to have little time to concern itself with the East. But go and do your duty. The sower seldom reaps. But if you succeed in passing on the Yoga of the body to only a few of your friends, you have done your duty to your brothers in the Occident. In any case, the teaching will only appeal to those whose mind is free from the blindness of materialism and whose spiritual world is open for a more beautiful and higher order of life . . . But remember, this is your most sacred duty.—When you receive a message from me, across the seas, you will know it is time for you to come home . . . that your native land is calling you . . . Go, my boy, Heaven be with you! . . ."

That is how I came to Europe.

II

— — — — —

What is Hatha Yoga ?

THE greatest miracle on earth is man.—His body consisting of bones, flesh and blood hides secrets he has been seeking for thousands of years to unravel, in the search for a solution to the great enigma, the great mystery of the great sphinx. Many have tried to solve this mystery of man, but only a few have been able to make the sphinx speak. Only the very rarest of seekers who delved deeper and deeper, untiringly, into their own SELF, finally succeeded in comprehending the greatest secret there is: themselves.

In India people have been studying the secrets of the human soul from time immemorial, and many have devoted their whole lives to this goal in order to discover: *what is man?—and what is his destiny here on earth?*

They withdrew from the commotion of the world and concentrated all their thoughts and desires on the one question: who am I?—Their indefatigable striving, the iron endurance and the yearning with which they pursued their search for truth—all bore fruit, and lo!—their spirit was enlightened, and spread out before them lay the whole secret of BEING. They understood LIFE. They were able to see the deepest, hiddenmost causes. And open before them, they saw the path which leads out of suffering, upwards to freedom, happiness, eternal bliss. . . . They knew that this state is attainable for every human being, and those who had been thus enlightened took pity on suffering mankind and began to teach people the way to redemption and liberation.

Various ways lead to the summit. Many will take the comfortable, easy serpentine path upward, because their physical constitution is not adapted to steep climbing.—Others will take a short-cut, climbing up more steeply.—And lastly, there are those who choose the shortest way, scaling the walls of rock in order to reach their goal sooner.

Similarly, man can approach his great inner goal by various paths, according to his spiritual and physical abilities. The great teachers have worked out several systems in order to make the self-appointed goal attainable for everybody. These systems shorten the path, and those who apply them reach their appointed goal faster and more easily.

The collective name for these systems is Yoga.

The great teachers and masters who have reached their goals by travelling the path of Yoga are called Yogis.

The various systems of Yoga differ only in their starting point. Their essence and their goal is always the same: perfect self-knowledge. This goal, however, can only be reached through unconditional self discipline. Hence, the various systems of Yoga first teach us self control. But there are Yoga systems which proceed by disciplining the mind; there are systems which begin with the control of the feelings; and there are others which take the body as the starting point, etc., according to the natural tendencies and abilities of the pupil. Corresponding to the different paths followed, the various Yogas have different names. It is recommended, however, to begin with that Yoga which starts with control of the body. This is the way of perfect health, and its name is HATHA YOGA.

The name Hatha Yoga goes back to the truth on which this system is founded. Our body is enlivened by positive and negative currents, and when these currents are in complete equilibrium, we enjoy perfect health. In the ancient language of the Orient, the positive current is designated by the letter 'HA' which is equivalent in meaning to 'SUN.' The negative current is called 'THA' meaning 'MOON.' The word YOGA has a double meaning. On the one hand, it is equivalent to 'joining' while the second meaning is 'yoke.' Thus 'HATHA YOGA' signifies the perfect knowledge of the two energies, the positive sun and negative moon energies, their joining in perfect harmony and complete equilibrium, and the ability to control their energies absolutely, that is, to bend them under the yoke of our 'SELF.'

20

This system is unique in the entire world, since it consciously perfects the body, compensates for any physical defects, and fills it with glowing life force. Hatha Yoga leads us back to nature, acquaints us with the healing forces dwelling in herbs, trees and roots, teaches us about our own body and the forces acting within it, and leads us to the close harmony of body and soul. The body reacts at the slightest impulses of the mind, and the state of the mind is powerfully influenced by the condition of the body. This reciprocal relationship is utilized by Hatha Yoga, and both mind and body are made healthy. The path to be followed is that of making our body and all its activities conscious. Even the sympathetic nervous system and all those organs whose functioning is usually independent of my consciousness can be made subservient to my will. The incalculable advantage of this is that any malfunctioning can be prevented, and the body can be saved from diseases which originate in functional causes. For example, I can control the activity of my heart and prevent it from palpitations resulting from an external stimulus like fright, bad news or sudden joy. Thus I can protect my heart from dilation, degeneration of the cardiac muscle, or other diseases. Or if I can control the secretions of my glandular system, I can govern the functions of almost all the organs of my body and thus govern my physical condition. The Hatha Yogi who has reached the highest level of ability has complete and absolute control over his body. He can regulate at will the activity of his heart, his digestive organs and the functioning of every other organ in his body. Countless travellers from the West who, after great difficulties, have had the good fortune to find a true Hatha Yogi during their visit to India have confirmed the fact that Yogis of 80 or 90 years give the impression of being 30 or 40, and that—by occidental standards—they live to an incredibly ripe old age because they can recharge their bodies with new life energies at will.

Merely prolonging their lives, however, is not the Yogis' goal. Hatha Yoga is not an end in itself, but rather a preparation for a higher spiritual Yoga. In a sick body it is very difficult to develop consciousness and quicken the mind to a higher level of activity. For this reason, we should first get acquainted with

21

the forces acting within our bodies in order to be able to use and control them properly later. Then our body is no longer an impediment during our climb up to higher mental and spiritual planes. Some persons are content to come into possession of magic powers with the aid of which they can perform things commonly regarded as miracles. Such people are stranded halfway to the goal and can make no progress. The goal we must strive for can only be this: liberation from the prison of the material world. Let us, therefore, not mistake the end for the means. The knowledge of our body and its secret powers is—no matter how important—still merely a means to an end. Hence a true Hatha Yogi will never make a display of his science and ability just to satisfy idle curiosity. Anyone who does so is no real Hatha Yogi. The true Hatha Yogi uses his abilities only when he can assist others through their use.

My own master, for example, never told us pupils what powers he could command. Once he was sitting in his little hut deep in the forest. In a clearing in the front of the hut, we pupils were engrossed in conversation. Suddenly a mongoose came out of a thicket. Half dead, the poor little creature dragged itself over the ground, and as it came nearer, we saw that it had been bitten by a snake. Its instinct drove it towards our teacher's hut. It was barely able to drag itself up to the door where it stopped and writhed in its death struggle. Our master laid his right hand on the little animal and fell into a trance. For a time he remained thus. Suddenly the mongoose quivered, shook itself and ran away again, fresh and well. Now we had *seen* what powers our master commanded.

In recent times occidental medical science has turned its attention towards Hatha Yoga, and those who know the secrets of Hatha Yoga—the Yogis—offer valuable information for the aims and ends of medical science.

The lower degree of Hatha Yoga is so interesting and useful that it is worth while getting acquainted with it and devoting our attention to it. Even the greatest masters had to begin their learning with this step, for without the alphabet there can be no reading. The first step of Hatha Yoga teaches us the art of being healthy!

First and foremost we must get acquainted with our body,

22

but not in theory as in the study of anatomy. Anatomy teaches us *what* is in the human body and *where* it is to be found. Really *knowing* my body, however, means something quite different. It means, assuming I know, for example, where my heart is, that I can also go down with my consciousness into my heart; that I can feel its shape, auricles, ventricles and valves—all so clearly and positively that this condition could perhaps best be expressed in the following way: 'I am my heart.' And I must be able to do the same with my stomach, intestines, liver, kidneys, and every fibre of my body. One who has never practised any Yoga exercises can, at most, know his palate and the inside of his mouth to this extent. One who wants to become a Hatha Yogi, however, must practise so long that he is able to direct his consciousness to the smallest parts of his body. When he reaches this point, the next step is to direct his consciousness, *united with his willpower*, to the minutest fibres of his body. To return to the previous example, it is no longer adequate to be able to penetrate my heart with my consciousness; but I must bring it under my authority. My heart must subordinate itself to my will, so that it can pump blood slower or faster as I see fit. This is not impossible! Just as anybody can learn to move his tongue, his fingers or many other parts of his body at will, anyone can also learn through systematic practice to control every part of the body. Even among average people, there are great differences in the extent to which their bodies are conscious. There are also differences according to profession. A pianist's fingers are much more independent and conscious than the fingers of a person who has never played the piano. Why?—because the pianist has made his fingers more conscious through constant exercise. The Hatha Yogi pupil also practises constantly, day after day, year after year, with patience and endurance. But he practises how to lead his consciousness into every part of his body. Is this worth while? Yes! For the result is worthy of admiration. He discovers secret forces in himself which, little by little, he learns to control. He learns that there are two life currents active in his body and that the complete equilibrium of these two forces means perfect health.

Simultaneously with the expansion of his consciousness, the

pupil comes to the realization that everything that lives in time and space is alive because it carries within itself polarity and rhythm. He begins to see the secrets of creation. In that moment when the creative principle leaves the absolute and splits in two, the negative and positive pole, i.e., polarity, is born. Between the two there arises a pulsating connection, rhythm is born, and there begins the manifestation of LIFE.

Even in crystals we can discover the presence of positive and negative poles, and we find them in all degrees of expressions of life. Polarity and rhythm give life to the entire universe. The movements of gigantic bodies in endless space, with their planets and satelites—even the sunspots, the throbbing heart-beats of living beings, our own breathing and being, all this occurs in a rhythm originating in polarity. Positive and negative currents alternate rhythmically, creating positive and negative conditions in complete equilibrium.

In Indian mythology the rhythm active throughout the universe is symbolized by the dancing figure of the god Shiva. The dance is a manifestation of rhythm.

Our earth, too, has two poles, and we humans who are born of dust and return to dust again also carry polarity within us, as positive and negative poles. The positive pole is in the top of the skull, at the spot where our hair forms a whorl. This point is easily located on a child's head. The negative pole is in the coccyx, the lowest vertebra. Between these two poles there is a current of extremely high frequency and short wave-length. This tension is LIFE!

The carrier of life is the spinal column.

Life wanted to manifest itself, and so it expanded the topmost vertebra of the spinal column and developed it into a skull. It formed the fine material in the latter into a conductor of a current and gave it the ability to express intelligence and feeling. Thus the brain came into existence. Through this material Life wanted to see, hear, smell, and feel. Thus the organs of sense evolved: eyes, ears, nose, mouth and sensory nerves. In order to move in space and be able to act, it created feet and hands. So that this creature could continue to exist and supply a replacement in case of deterioration, it created the various organs for reproduction and propagation. The nervous system

24

serves to transmit the life current. Finally, this vehicle of life, moving about on two feet, was given a name: 'MAN.' LIFE within man became conscious of itself and, consequently, it spoke and said, 'I AM.'

LIFE within us is what man refers to as 'I' within himself. LIFE is the 'I', the ever-living, immortal SELF that was never born and can never die, for the SELF is LIFE and LIFE cannot die. It is only the body that is born and will die. But the body is only the clothing, the outer garment of the SELF, an instrument by which it manifests itself on the material plane.

When LIFE becomes conscious of itself and leads back this consciousness, via the intelligence, into its own SELF, we call this condition CONSCIOUSNESS OF SELF.

The SELF clothed itself with the body and by means of the nervous system it radiates itself, that is LIFE, into every fibre of the body, filling the latter with perfect equilibrium and harmony. Thus the functioning of the body is regular, that is, HEALTHY.

Man carries within himself the positive-sending and at the same time the negative-receiving—resisting characteristics of his being. Within his personality which is woven of contrasts he must preserve complete balance, join the opposites together, supplementing each by the other, and reconcile them within himself. Only then is he perfect. Only then is he whole and healthy and able to perform his earthly task, just as complementary colours supplement each other in sunlight: red and green—violet and yellow—blue and orange. These colours are direct opposites, yet for that very reason, they belong together. Their unity results in perfection. The laws of spirit and body involve the same direct opposition. The law of the spirit is selflessness, whereas that of the body is selfishness. And yet man must learn to join the two in complete harmony and to manifest them in himself. This truth was taught by all prophets and great teachers who ever lived on earth, for they knew the secret of being: the tension between the positive and the negative pole. For this reason they all used the same symbol to represent the absolute commander of the opposing forces—the God-Man who attained perfection. In every religion this symbol was the same—a six-pointed star made by interweaving two triangles.

25

This star symbolizes the secret of the forces which maintain the universe, and at the same time also the perfected being which is master of life and manifests spirit and matter in the same way: the man who has perfected creation within himself; that is: the God-Man.

The God-Man does not use the body as an end in itself, but as a vehicle for manifesting the spirit: UNSELFISH LOVE, and he fills his body uniformly with the highest energies. His body is therefore enlivened with consciousness.

The consciousness of the average man is still on a very low level of development. For that reason, the radiation of the life current within his body is only conscious to a very low degree; for the most part unconscious, automatic. The body of a person on such a low level of development is much less alive than that of a person on a more advanced plane. The latter has many more convolutions of the brain. His nervous system is much more closely woven, that is, more conscious, more alive, and as a consequence, his body is a much more willing and elastic vehicle for his SELF.

The bodily movements of the conscious person with a very live body are different from those of a person on a lower level of development. The movements of the more conscious person we characterise as 'graceful', 'supple' and 'beautiful', while we refer to someone in whose body the expressions of LIFE stand on a lower level as 'clumsy' or 'awkward'. We feel a thing to be beautiful or charming in which LIFE expresses itself more maturely; that is, we discover and recognize in it the universal SELF, our own BEING.

The only bliss that exists is *to find oneself*! That is what we are seeking in every joy, in every feeling of happiness. If our SELF is in this condition, if it rests within itself, there is a complete equilibrium in the life forces we radiate. In this case, our mind and our body are both healthy.

In persons on a lower level, the equilibrium can be easily upset through ignorance or as a result of inadequate consciousness. Such persons fall out of their SELF, because the unconscious part of their person is bigger than the conscious part. This disturbance to their equilibrium also expresses itself in their way of thinking and in their spiritual life. The result is

26

that the balance between positive and negative currents is disturbed. If, however, there is not a perfect balance between the two life energies radiated, there develops the condition we call sickness.

A major prerequisite for health is, therefore, that of gradually expanding our consciousness and leading it into all parts of our body. In this way we can avoid disturbing the order—we can prevent disease. And if sickness is already present we consciously and intentionally restore the condition of order.

This is what is taught by the science and art known as HATHA YOGA.

III

— — — — —

Every Disease Has Mental Causes

"I AM the way, the truth and the life," we read in the Bible. This same fact is taught by Indian Yogis: LIFE is the SELF.

In its true nature, the SELF is shining, perfect, spotlessly pure and without sin. But when it took on material form—a body—it acquired the sin of matter, the sin of the world. The fact of being dependent on matter and time lowered its consciousness, and it required a development of millions of years for the physical body to become conscious again. Even today this development is not yet finished, as the consciousness of the average person is still far from expanding and uniting with his own supreme, divine SELF. Mankind, like a great body, has travelled along this path of development, and thus each historical age shows a certain degree of progress. However, there are always individuals who are below the average level of development, and others who stand above it. There are no two people whose degree of consciousness is equal. Only people who have reached perfection are equal, only those whose consciousness has reached and united with the universal SELF. Only such persons think completely alike. However, even they still bear the stamp of their individual filter, their body. Only in essentials, in spirit, are they one.

The manifold events of a lifetime, the infinite interplay of human destinies, cause differing experiences and influences. As a result, human consciousness develops in different ways. In one individual the experiences and impressions are brought by the consciousness to a higher stage of progress in the very field in which, in another individual, they are degenerating. However, it is possible that in some other direction of develop-

28

ment the first of these individuals is behind while the second has made considerable progress. These infinite variations in the degree of consciousness we have attained are the cause of the fact that there are as many different individualities as there are people.

The SELF, this eternal spring of LIFE, in complete equilibrium and perfect harmony, uniformly radiates the energy of life into the body. If a person's consciousness is equally developed in every direction, even if it is on a low level, life energy will flow uniformly into his body. The positive and negative currents function in equilibrium, and his body is well. The condition of consciousness of the individual acts as a filter which distributes the radiated life energy into the various mental and nervous centres which the India Yogis call chakras. When for any reason the consciousness departs from a uniform, balanced development, either through evolving one-sidedly in a certain direction, or through being retarded in another, there is a shift in the flow of life forces, and the equilibrium ceases. However, the radiation of the supreme SELF with its perfect balance endeavours to smooth out irregularities, and with tremendous strength it forces its way past the irregular distribution of energy. This levelling out of irregularities, this struggle for the re-establishment of order, is the condition people call sickness.

Health is the natural and prerequisite condition for the body. Life force in mankind is not only dependent upon the conscious will to live, but also active as subconscious life instinct. Life instinct manifests itself in two ways—as the instinct for self preservation and the instinct for the preservation of the species. Both of these are tremendous, world-moving primitive forces. The urge for the preservation of the species ensures continuity when the means of manifestation, the body, is worn out. It provides for replacement through generating descendants. On the other hand, the instinct of self preservation strives to maintain the life of the individual being as long as possible. Nature strives powerfully to maintain the health we have, and if we do not sin against her laws, we can retain our health, undisturbed, until we die. " Nature never wanted man to leave his body before advanced old age," said Ramacharaka, "and if only everybody would obey the laws of nature from his child-

29

hood on, instead of constantly working against them, the death of human beings through disease in their youth or middle age would be as rare as death by violence."

Life force is constantly active in us. It provides the equilibrium. It smooths out irregularities and preserves our health, and all this despite the fact that mankind, day after day, defiantly tramples under foot the golden rules of healthy living. The urge for self preservation has only one purpose—and there can be no argument about it—this urge demands LIFE and HEALTH! It is so strong that, in moments of danger, it makes the meekest person into a wild beast. Countless times have we read that people on a sinking ship choked and trampled each other in order to get into a lifeboat, while only those with a highly developed spiritual life who had already reached the point of impersonality were so unselfish as to be able to fight down the instinct for self preservation. This powerful force is working within us ceaselessly day after day to preserve our health and offset the mistakes we make. It sets in motion a great house-cleaning process to free our organism from the poisonous wastes and toxins which have accumulated through our negligence.

Life Force puts the urge for self preservation in the service of our health. Ramacharaka said of it: " This works within us independently of our will—like the needle of a compass which, no matter how we may turn the instrument out of its natural position, constantly points towards the north pole, towards health". In vain do we disobey, in vain do we turn away from it; for it lives on in us nevertheless and acts without interruption. The same force draws the delicate shoot out of the seed and often forces it through a layer that is a thousand times harder, all in order for the tiny stems to reach the sunshine. The same force causes the young slip to grow upwards towards the sky and its roots to spread out in the earth. If an open wound is made on our body, this wound is healed by life force with astonishing accuracy and with a perfection man himself could never attain. *Medicus curat, natura sanat*, said our fathers quite rightly. The physician wields the operating knife, sews up the wound, and creates the prerequisites for healing. The rest is left to nature. If a man breaks a leg, the doctor sets the bones, but the healing process itself is provided by life force. If the latter is unable to develop its full strength in our interest, it is still far from giving up the struggle. Instead, it adapts itself to the circumstances in order to be able to help us at such time and place as this becomes possible again. If we give life force a free hand, it keeps us in perfect health. Even if we suppress it through an unintelligent and unnatural way of living, it does not cease to act on our behalf. Even under inhibiting circumstances, it always endeavours to help us, despite our ingratitude and ignorance. Up to the moment of our death, life force is fighting to maintain the health of our body. Its adaptability is almost limitless. A seed falls into a tiny crack, yet splits the boulder asunder, or—if the rock is too strong—climbs out of the narrow slit up into the air and sunshine. Whatever the circumstances, life must conquer.

A living organism does not get sick as long as it lives according to the primitive rules of nature. Health is nothing else than a life under natural conditions. Disease, on the other hand, is a result of unnatural living. To our sorrow, modern civilization forces us into an unnatural way of living, so that life force can only protect our health to a limited extent. We neither eat, nor drink, nor sleep, nor breathe, nor clothe ourselves properly and naturally.

Hatha Yoga teaches us how to utilize, store and promote the free flow of life force to the maximum extent. Whoever follows the rules of Hatha Yoga will never be sick and will enjoy complete health until old age. One of the most important prerequisites, however, is to get acquainted with all manifestations of life force and to learn how these can be developed and shaped—in a word—how we can put these energies to work for our consciousness.

Man is spirit clothed in flesh. Within himself he reflects the laws of both the spirit and the body. The flow of life energy manifests itself in mankind—from the absolute, spiritual SELF down to the material plane, the body—on every level. The energy which manifests itself on the spiritual plane nearest to the SELF is positive. The energy farthest from the SELF, that is, the energy which quickens the body, is negative. The positive energy is life-giving, and negative energy is life-receiving and conducting. As long as the two energies are in equilibrium, the individual is mentally and physically well; but as soon as he directs his consciousness one-sidedly towards the spiritual or the physical plane, he has opened the door for the various kinds of irregularities. We know from experience that people who do constant mental work exclusively are always of a rather weak and delicate physical constitution. The positive forces expand at the expense of the negative, and such a body has little resistance. However, if such a person, through consciously conducted exercises of Hatha Yoga, directs his consciousness, at least for a few minutes daily, towards those nervous centres which are called upon to supply the body with life force, the balance is restored; his body is strengthened, and his resistance increases.

It is likewise an unhealthy condition and one which promotes susceptibility to many kinds of suffering, when a person goes to the other extreme and directs his consciousness primarily towards the material plane, showing interest only in heavy eating and drinking. The preponderance of the physical side—obesity and mental obtuseness—are the consequences of such an upset in the individual's equilibrium. These are simple examples for the one-sided unbalancing of the consciousness towards one extreme or the other. In these cases the individual shifts the mental and material planes in their relation to each other. However, it is also possible to sin against the proper relationship if each plane is regarded all alone, separately, by itself.

A person can manifest the creative force individually, in every degree, from the spiritual plane to the material plane, as positive and negative energy. He is balanced if he utilizes his powers in the proper manner, i.e., inwardly negative and outwardly positive. We call such a person positive according to his outward manifestation. These people are the creative leaders who are able to make something out of nothing, spreading life and fruitfulness all around. Such persons utilize their positive and negative spiritual energies in the proper relationship: inwardly, in the direction of the divine radiation, they are negative, they receive. They accept intuition, believe in themselves, and have faith in their own SELF. Outwardly they are positive: they give, they create, they produce. Likewise on the plane of their mind

32

and emotions, they are in balance and healthy. Radiating joy, sunshine, confidence, love, kindness, and warmth, they are positive in their outward manifestations; however, at the proper time, they are also negative, as they accept the love that radiates towards themselves. Such people are also physically healthy, for their life energy—the combustion within the body—is in equilibrium with the resistance, with the matter composing the body.

If we utilize our forces in the opposite way, our body will sooner or later fall sick. People make this mistake even on the mental plane. They do not believe in a higher SELF that gives life to their person. Instead of opening the way for the eternal source of strength dwelling within their soul, they lock the door through their doubts, drop away from their own SELF and suffer a lack of self confidence. Such a person always looks elsewhere for help, he is powerless and helpless, he is afraid of everything and sees evil everywhere. Instead of radiating creative power and being active in a constructive way, he ruins his whole life through his disbelief. He fails where others succeed. This kind of person is like a vacuum into which everything falls and disappears. That is the negative individual!—a dark gorge, a bottomless pit into which every good human effort falls, a negative force that absorbs and completely neutralizes every bit of positive energy with which it comes into contact. Let us ever be on our guard against such a fate! The mistake begins with the words: "I never succeed at anything!" Woe be unto us if we ever make such a statement! In so doing, we set up a wall before our own sources of power—a wall that we can only tear down again with the greatest effort. We must never be negative. When someone wants to undertake a good and useful thing, let us guard ourselves against ever discouraging him, saying "You won't succeed anyway!" No! We will succeed if we believe in what we are doing and approach it rightly, if we have enough self-confidence to be able to master the difficulties. Let us have confidence in our SELF which has built up our body independently of our consciousness, this wonderful instrument, this magnificent vehicle that fulfils all its purposes, and let us believe that this marvellous constructive force is still dwelling within us in the depths of our SELF. And why not! We are alive, and this means that our SELF is there, and if we open the door with our faith, it helps us to build up our destiny as magnificently and purposefully as our body; it also helps us to salvage the things we have bungled.

The negative individual expects help from outside not from within. He is selfish and has neither understanding for others nor for himself. He is morose, despondent, peevish and complains constantly. He has no love, but expects others to love him. Even in this he is negative. He does not know what true love is. He only knows passion. What he thinks is love is nothing else but desire for something or somebody. The energies utilized in this incorrect fashion disturb his mental equilibrium. Through the circuit of the nervous system, the mind directly affects the body. If our minds get out of balance, this causes such strong shocks and fluctuations that the nerves are shattered. However, since the work of the bodily organs is guided and controlled by the nerves, this impairs the health of all the organs of the body.

From his own experience everyone realizes the close connection between the functioning of his organism and the fluctuations of the emotions. Even the healthiest person can suffer certain physical changes through receiving bad news, even though no one has so much as laid a finger on his body. He loses his appetite, gets a headache, or develops other unpleasant symptoms. Terror can cause him to blanch, the blood to leave his head, and his body to fall in a faint. As a condition of consciousness, terror develops a surplus of negative current, so that order is disturbed in the currents of the body, and a negative condition results. If an individual becomes angry, blood rushes to his head, and he gets palpitations of the heart. This is the reverse of the conditions described above: positive currents predominate, and a one-sidedly positive condition appears. Every similar disturbance is connected with unpleasant symptoms, but generally the individual's natural defences are able to set up order again quickly. However, if bad effects are repeated in short intervals or if they continue, a serious disturbance in the order of currents occurs sooner or later, and the result is DISEASE!

The one-sided development of consciousness, or the stagnation of the latter, can also be the cause of numerous serious diseases, nervous disturbances and even of mental diseases. Our body and our mind are healthy when the positive current of life force manifesting itself on the material plane—in our body—is in perfect equilibrium with the negative force: the force of resistance of the body. In such a condition, there is a balance between the life force and the resistance of the body which carries it. In an individual on a low level of consciousness, the tension of the life force streaming into his body is low. His nervous system is adjusted to a corresponding resistance. With the expansion of consciousness, the tension of life force increases and consequently the power of resistance of the nervous system must also increase. If this is done step by step in complete equilibrium, the nervous system has time to strengthen itself, parallel with the increasing tension of life currents, and to develop a corresponding resistance. If, however, the development takes place haphazardly, in fits and starts, the nervous system becomes ill due to the strong currents and sudden changes for which it is not prepared because it has not been able to build up the required resistance. This situation is similar to that prevailing when too much electricity is switched into a circuit. When this happens, the wire, i.e., the resistance, burns out. The resistance against the life current is the nervous system which becomes disordered if exposed to a sudden and excessively strong current. Functional disorders occur, and inflammations and even complete paralysis are possible. The disturbance occurring in the consciousness causes various mental diseases.

The purpose of Yoga is to make our human consciousness dependent upon our will, to expand it systematically, intentionally, from one step to another, and at the same time, to increase and strengthen the resistance of the circuit which carries the constantly growing life energy, i.e., the nervous system. Thus the final goal is: divine consciousness developed to perfection and its perfect manifestation in the body: the God-Man! The Hindus call persons who have climbed to this level of perfection 'Jivan Mukti.'

This is the sense and purpose of our life. Destiny, with all the experiences and troubles it brings, likewise causes a constant expansion of our consciousness. But as we constantly grope in darkness, we pay for our ignorance, and the unequal distribution of forces allows thousands of different diseases to come upon us.

Inasmuch as diseases always arise from the fact that one of the two life currents has the upper hand over the other, we divide them into two major groups, positive and negative diseases.

If we overstrain the body's life force, either through exaggerated sexuality or through excessive mental work, this causes increased combustion. The body is exhausted and falls into a negative condition. Its resistance is too low. Such negative diseases are tuberculosis, chronic inflammations, allergic disorders, stomach and intestinal ulcers, etc. Convalescence, neurasthenia and depressions are also negative conditions.

The opposite happens when for any reason, life energy is reduced or withdrawn so that the cells of the body, lacking a concentrated force, start to go wild, forming tumours and cancerous growths. The result is likewise a negative condition of the body, but the cause is to be sought in the opposite side, not as in the case of tuberculosis or in the morbific agents of allergy. This is also the reason why people who incline toward allergies are very seldom predisposed to cancer.

Positive diseases, by and large, are those acute disorders accompanied by a high fever, i.e., inflammations, such as pneumonia, tonsilitis, nephritis, or neuralgia, and those types of infectious diseases which are also associated with high fever, such as typhus and scarlet fever.

There are mixed diseases in which the positive and negative conditions alternate, as in malaria for example, or in the presence of pus in the body, when fever temperatures running over 100°F alternate with subnormal temperatures.

The organism is constantly striving to effect a balance. If, for example, our body gets into a negative condition as a result of over-cooling and if it becomes defenceless against bacteria, the organism immediately develops a large quantity of positive currents—for self protection—and the body's condition becomes positive: we run a high fever. The sudden predominance of positive currents causes plethora and inflammations. The latter, however, destroys the bacilli which accumulated during the

36

negative condition, and little by little, the balance is restored.

During the course of serious inflammatory diseases, after the bacteria are destroyed and the over-induction of positive current is no longer necessary, a sudden shift occurs to the negative condition, the temperature drops below normal, and the patient, although the actual disease is overcome, falls into a critical condition as a result of the abrupt transitionless change of currents. In such cases, we give the patient black coffee or some other stimulant. After positive diseases, there is normally a negative condition, the period of convalescence. After swinging far out to the right, the pendulum swings equally far to the left and only little by little comes back to the normal oscillation, which corresponds to its own length, that is to its own period. This is also true of human beings. If we get too much of any kind of energy, more than is suited to our personality, this causes a strong reaction, and the equilibrium is only gradually restored.

However, if we consciously prevent the first irregular outward swing of the pendulum, the sickness does not occur at all.

Let us take an example: Supposing my body is suddenly and unexpectedly cooled. If the blind laws of nature are allowed to operate within me, my body's condition turns negative. The bacteria increase. Nature defends herself against them and develops more positive power. Fever occurs, and the sickness runs its natural course.

If, however, when the sudden cooling first hits my body, I simultaneously, intentionally, develop correspondingly more positive force and lead this force into my body, this immediately restores the equilibrium, the bacteria do not increase, and thus no fever is necessary. I have prevented the disease!

That is Yoga!

We have already seen the physical changes that can be caused by simple fright if, even for only a short time, any force predominates over the others. Regardless of whether the over-balance of any kind of energy arises through a lasting mental disturbance or from a constant mental condition, this causes grave physical changes and serious diseases. This fact has been proved by the research of Western psychiatrists. Rage, fear, grief, sorrow, fright, jealousy, despondency, pessimism, and similar negative impulses undermine the health, destroy the nervous system and lower the resistance of the whole organism, making it more susceptible to disease and delaying the healing process.

As early as 1879 the American professor of medicine, Dr. Gates, published the results of his experience in this field. He drew off his patient's breath into an ice-cooled glass tube, thus causing it to condense. Under normal breathing, the 'rhodopsin-iodide' did not cause any appreciable deposit. Five minutes later, however, when the patient was angry, there was a brownish deposit in the tube, indicating that, after the sudden emotional surge, there was a certain chemical product in the patient's breath. If this substance was extracted and injected in a human being or an animal, it provoked great excitement. Profound grief, such as that caused by loss of a dearly beloved child, produced a grey deposit.

"In the course of my experience and experiments", writes Doctor Gates, "I came to the conviction, that irate, angry and despondent emotional states cause harmful, poisonous products in the organism, while the good feelings—contentment, happiness, jollity, good spirits, love—and good thoughts, mobilize the healing powers of the organism. Among the negative emotions, fear and despair are perhaps the most destructive for the nervous system." According to Horace Fletcher, fear fills us with noxious carbon dioxide and poisons our atmosphere. It causes a mental, spiritual and moral choking, very often a slow death.

"Actually, medical science records many cases in which people with sensitive nervous systems collapsed lifeless in mortal fear, as if they had been struck by lightning. A very interesting report is provided by a professor of medicine in Australia: 'The greatest danger that can threaten a growing child is the imposition of its mother's nervous fears. Nervous young mothers try to protect their youngsters from every draught and forbid everything that would tend to teach them courage, endurance, and self-confidence. Such mothers pour into their children a slow-working poison and do them lifelong harm. We should raise our children so that they do not know what fear is. That is the most beautiful, most valuable heritage we can give them. . . .'"

Instead, children are taught to fear the bow-wow and the devil. In every language there is an appropriate expression. In all parts of the world, children are frightened by their parents and teachers, so that they will not do this or that. A destructive mechanism begins to operate on the child's mind. The principle of auto-suggestion—which is very little known and vastly underrated in the Occident—gives the child a mental handicap and when it grows up, it will be oppressed by fright, fear, inferiority complexes, and moral, sexual, and professional inhibitions.

Eighty per cent of humanity is afraid. Fear of sickness, poverty, and misfortune; worry about losing loved ones; fear of death and finally fear of fear itself.

How many people ruin their own lives and those of their relatives through being afraid of the morrow and because, by reason of this fear, they dare not grant themselves physical or mental rest. They are afraid of the lean years that are perhaps yet to come. Most people are constantly preparing for evil and collecting and saving like busy ants. Their children must suffer and do without just as they do, so that someday, thirty or forty years hence, 'the little family home' will be together. The unhealthy way of living, and the lack of mental and physical recuperation lasting throughout decades, avenges itself implacably. With a stomach disorder, arterio-sclerosis or a heart disorder, the individual can profit little from his country home and his bank deposits.

The great world teacher, Jesus Christ, who came out of the East tells us in magnificent words how both body and mind can be kept healthy:

" Take no thought for your life, what ye shall eat, or what ye shall drink; nor yet for your body, what ye shall put on. Is not the life more than meat, and the body than raiment? Behold the fowls of the air: for they sow not, neither do they reap, nor gather into barns; yet your heavenly Father feedeth them.

" Are ye not much better than they? Which of you by taking thought can add one cubit unto his stature? And why take ye thought for raiment? Consider the lilies of the field, how they grow; they toil not, neither do they spin: And yet I say unto you, that even Solomon in all his glory was not arrayed like one of these. Wherefore, if God so clothe the grass of the field, which today is, and tomorrow is cast into the oven, shall he not much more clothe you, O ye of little faith? Therefore take no thought, saying, What shall we eat? or, What shall we drink? or, Wherewithal shall we be clothed? For after all these things do the Gentiles seek: for your heavenly Father knoweth that ye have need of all these things. But seek ye first the kingdom of God, and his righteousness; and all these things shall be added unto you. Take therefore no thought for the morrow: for the morrow shall take thought for the things of itself. Sufficient unto the day is the evil thereof."

Probably no one has ever expressed the basic rule of Hatha Yoga so magnificently: A mental serenity which knows no fear, outward thoughtfulness, and the philosophy of the religious man, who places his unqualified trust in the higher order of powers and who knows how to control his emotions.

Hatha Yoga exercises have a wonderful effect on the struggle against fear. They give one the basis of physical self control. We must know that the body reacts to every mental impulse. Primarily, this is done by the nervous system and the internal ductless glandular system which is so highly developed for the preservation of life and which is of decisive importance from the point of view of the nervous system and the protection of life.

Dr. Lorand and Dr. Sajous have shown that the various vegetative functions depend primarily on the condition of the internal-secretion glands which have no ducts and which pour their secretions directly into the blood. If this activity is diminished, the result is disease, premature old age and finally death. Thus the emotions and passions, through their destructive effect on the endocrine glands, are the implacable enemies of health.

The most important ductless glands are the thyroid, pineal, pituitary, suprarenal, and sexual glands.

Emotional crises have the effect of increasing the blood pressure through the latter's regulatory mechanism, the suprarenal capsule. This explains the fact that persons with a quick temper suffer from early arterio-sclerosis and frequent disturbances in the blood stream. According to the Scientific Laboratory for Yoga Research in Lonavla, India, as well as

Occidental medical science, constant despondency and melancholy have such an effect on the thyroid gland that myxoedema, a disease similar to exophthalmic goitre (Basedow's disease) can be caused. The thyroid glands in the throat are protective devices of the first order put there by nature as a defence against various kinds of poisonings. Degenerate thyroid glands cause many kinds of disease, premature old age and early death. On the other hand, if the thyroid gland functions regularly under a happy frame of mind, we can keep our body elastic and buoyant far into a ripe old age. Emotional states have the strongest effect on the hypothesis of the brain and on the pineal gland, as has been proved by Dr. Sajous experimentally. Professor Pel, after great emotional disturbances, was able to find cases of acromegaly.

The system of ductless glands plays a particularly important part in Yoga, as these glands are the location of certain centres of consciousness which the Yogis call 'chakras'. These chakras are a connecting link between mind and body. If we know the role these chakras play in the distribution of force and storing of energy, then we know the kind of reaction which the maintaining of a mental condition will cause in the body by acting on the ductless glands. In this way we can get acquainted with the more intimate relationship between various mental conditions and the different organs of the body, and thus we can gain control over the body. Here are a few examples. Experience and psychological research have shown that the formation of calculus (gallstones, kidney stones, etc.) is generally preceded by a long period of worry and sorrow. Sudden fright causes diarrhoea. Protracted fear and worry cause chronic intestinal catarrh. Frequent excitement paves the way for heart trouble and varicose veins. Disappointed hope or unsatisfied yearning causes an acid stomach and makes us susceptible to stomach ulcers. Protracted fear of death permanently impairs the function of the sexual glands. Characteristic of this is the fact that during the persecutions of the Jews—according to the experience of my pupils—Jewish women generally ceased to menstruate. It was believed that this was the result of their being fed a secret drug with sterilizing effects. Later during protracted sieges of many cities, Christian women who had been living under the agonizing fear of death, developed the same symptoms. The fear of death thus had merely acted as a wise governor valve of nature. Nature does not want any progeny as long as highly inhibiting conditions of life continue. Among men, the same cause resulted in impotence or a great lessening of the sexual urge. According to our experience, these general symptoms likewise disappeared when the fear of death ceased. Among the men, the pendulum then swung to the opposite extreme. In this way, nature restores the equilibrium, both of the individual as well as the race.

Excessive sensuality predisposes to tuberculosis. For this reason the susceptibility to tuberculosis is greatest during puberty. The over-excited condition of the sexual glands communicates itself to the other ductless glands with which it works in series, then to all other glands and to the hilar lymph nodes in the lungs. The stimulated condition of the hilar lymph nodes makes the lung over-sensitive and causes catarrh. In this way, the resistance of the lung is greatly reduced, so that it cannot fight off infection. The organism, in order to protect itself, spurs the glandular system on to greater activity, the individual becomes erotically even more excited, and his condition deteriorates.

In Hatha Yoga schools experience has shown that when a patient succeeds in disciplining his thoughts, he can, without any violent suppression, live in complete continence, parallel to the treatment he is getting. Thus, in very many seemingly hopeless cases, healing can be attained. Western physicians have also recognized a connection between tuberculosis and excessive sexuality. They suppose, however, that the erotic condition is the result of tuberculosis, whereas actually the opposite is true. People who are over sensual are thus more disposed to tuberculosis. If occidental medical science would compile statistics on the mental condition which precedes various diseases, it would soon realize the truth of what Hatha Yogis teach, namely, that *all disorders, even infectious diseases, are the result of mental causes.*

Western physicians shake their heads and talk about bacteria. As long as 6,000 years ago, Hatha Yogis in India knew that the immediate cause of disease was bacteria. True enough, they

42

had no microscopes. But they knew what a bacterium was and that it can successfully attack only those whose resistance is lowered or who are susceptible to this disease. Both of these conditions, however, are the result of an improper mental attitude. The Hatha Yogis who many thousands of years ago created the Indian medical science known as the Ayurveda, wrote on dried and specially prepared palm leaves:

'. . . The precipitating causes of diseases are myriads of tiny, invisible creatures. These together are nothing other than the body of the evil spirit. They can only attack a person who himself opens a breach in his own soul'. It is remarkable that the great European master Paracelsus taught something very similar: 'The best protection against every disease is a noble mind'.—The basic thought is the same.

I have been greatly surprised at the following experience. While on the one hand, recognized internes shake their heads at the oriental claim that even infectious diseases are due to mental causes and that disturbances of menstruation can be put right through treatment of the mind, there is a group of physicians who are equally active in trying to prove that mind and body are closely connected and that the condition of the mind is of decisive importance for health. These latter are the *psychologists*. In the books of world famous psychologists I have come across opinions which completely agree with that of the Yogis. I quote passages from the book 'The Mind is Everything' by the world-renowned specialist on nerves and hypnotism, Dr. Franz Volgesi:

'The sixty-eight cases of hypnotic action studied by Dr. Robert Heilig and Hans Holff prove that, with the aid of mental stimuli, serological, self-healing, and other changes can be caused within the organism. They are changes which cannot be 'consciously' simulated by the patient, as their course and control require the most precise technical knowledge and the utilization of special instruments. All authors agree that their research proves that every reaction of the organism intended for self-protection, including the *readiness to fight off bacilli and infectious material, is demonstrably dependent upon the mental condition.* In individuals who suffered from mental depressions, and in all others who were healthy but who were post-hypnotically induced into a state of mental depression, the blood's ability to defend itself (agglutination) against typhus bacilli was obviously reduced. The blood was likewise altered in its opsonic action against coli, streptococci and staphylococci. When patients were subjected to auto-suggestion leading towards a happy state of mind, the control experiments all showed increased possibilities for self protection. *In other words, the mental influences, within certain human limits, are effective with greater force than chemical, medical, and toxic effects'.*

Can there be a more striking proof for the claim of the Yogis in the Orient?

Even in the West it has been observed that some people are not susceptible to disease. They are immune. This means that in the individual concerned the positive and negative currents are in complete equilibrium and that the resistance of such persons is adequate for any attack. Hatha Yogis *do not conquer bacteria with chemicals.* They know that it is useless to kill bacteria if the patient's resistance remains low; for as long as this condition prevails, the bacteria will multiply again or else another pathogenic agent will appear and attack the organism. As long as this goes on, the disease never ends. Yogis prevent the disease through maintaining the equilibrium of currents, or if this has been disturbed and a disease is already present, they restore the balance between the two currents. In this way, the organism conquers the disease *through its own power and returns to permanent health.* The balance between the two currents is perfect when our mental equilibrium is perfect. Therefore, we must begin by setting the mind in order.

If I bite into a hard crust of bread and break a tooth, does this have a mental cause? Yes!

Through the nervous system the mind penetrates into the body. The nervous system directly affects the glandular system. Hence the production of hormones within the system of ductless glands depends directly on the mental condition of the individual. We know very well that the calcium or lime content of our bones—and consequently the hardness and resilience of our teeth—depends on the quantity and quality of the hormones circulating in our blood. If a tooth is decayed and brittle, this likewise has mental causes!

44

But how about accidents? If someone falls down a stairway and lands at the bottom, battered and bruised, does this also have mental causes?—Yes! But these causes lie deep below the conscious mind.

Every accident is a self-punishment of the individual. Every decision, every act, every movement has its point of origin within us. If someone who has gone up and down a stairway a hundred times, makes an awkward movement just this once and trips, there are inner causes at work. Dormant in the mind, a force antithetical to the purpose in view causes—by means of the nervous system—an improper reflex movement and—the accident happens. It is purely self-punishment!

Whoever realizes that every accident represents self-punishment, will ask himself, when he bumps his elbow or bites his tongue: 'Why has this happened?'—and instantly he hears the answer from out of the depths of his consciousness. . . .

There are people who are constantly bumping into things, stumbling at every other step, running into the corners of every cupboard. A thorough investigation of such an individual's mind reveals the causes, and when his mind is set in order, he returns to physical health, free from further accidents.

Let us not forget that we make our every movement; we—and nobody else—take our every step.—If I set my foot down beside the step instead of on it, if I raise my foot higher or less high than usual, or if in making a movement, I make a bigger swing or move more to the right or to the left—all these things have their causes within myself. It may happen that there is a long time-lag between cause and effect. It is possible that, years ago, I did or said something wrong that has been stored up under my conscious mind, waiting for an opportunity to manifest itself as an inappropriate—negative—movement. The Overself does not forget! At the proper moment it metes out punishment. It punishes through ourselves. It utilizes our thoughtlessness or a moment of danger when we have no time to reflect and must act *instinctively*. The pent up, selfish—isolating—forces avenge themselves upon us in such moments; they produce a movement which harms us instead of the one we would like to make which would do us good.

Even primitive man knew about these relationships; but he

45

did not know that he was judging himself and causing a punishing movement. Instead, he trembled before the manifestation of an unknown force and said: 'The punishment of God'! For the Yogi, however, the secret of his SELF lies spread out before him and he realizes that a powerful law dwelling within the depths of his own being has operated. Modern psychology has also come to the point of discovering the world which lies behind the conscious mind—that is, in the subconscious—and is now beginning to analyse its laws.

The law of the superior SELF active within us not only means that I myself cause all my illnesses and accidents, but it also includes the supremely comforting corollary that—if I utilize my energies properly—each of my movements and decisions will be for my own good. The individual whose mind is in equilibrium will always make the motion which is the most appropriate, the best for him. He will not allow any dross to build up an INSULATING WALL between his personality and his higher SELF, and therefore, in moments of peril, he will be able to rise to the highest plane. His ear is open for inner inspiration and, like a person who is all-knowing or illumined, he seizes the one possibility that will save him from danger.

What do we mean by 'proper utilization of our energies'?

When my acts are always motivated by impersonal, unselfish LOVE based on the universal SELF, my mind will be peaceful, balanced and healthy.

This, however, is the prerequisite for my also being physically healthy.

The prevention and healing of disease must therefore begin in the mind. And here we encounter the important role of the interrelationship of MIND and *body*. Hatha Yoga bases its system on this relationship and develops, in parallel, the individual's abilities and physical health.

From the very start this system eliminates the mistake under which occidental medical science is so woefully suffering, namely, that of healing the *diseases* instead of the *patient*!

Hatha Yoga teaches: Inasmuch as *we ourselves have caused our sicknesses, we must heal our abused body ourselves*! The teacher—whom Indian Yogis call 'Guru'—helps us find the cause, but *we must attain health by our own efforts.*

46

Hatha Yoga teaches us how to keep order among the forces which animate our body and—in case we have sinned against our health through unnatural living—how we can restore our physical wellbeing again. The ailing individual is a burden on himself and his fellows, and therefore the basic thesis of Hatha Yoga is:

TO BE HEALTHY IS A DUTY!

IV

— — — — —

Our Greatest Mistake:
WE CANNOT BREATHE!

ON the seventh day of my sojourn in Chitoor Forest I learnt the greatest truth of Hatha Yoga. Seven years later, however, when I observed the living habits of my European brethren, I noticed that their breathing consisted only of light shallow breaths corresponding to the lowest stage of life.

The Bible teaches us, that man without breath would be only a lifeless lump of earth, for God created man from earth and breathed into his nostrils the breath of life. Through this breath, i.e., respiration, Adam awoke to life.

The Vedanta philosophy tells us the same thing, when it says 'Without breathing there is no life on earth'.

Life means rhythm!—With its first breath the new-born baby enters into the rhythm of life; with its inhalation and exhalation, it begins to experience the flow of life in its alternating positive and negative phases, pulsating within it like an alternating current. Life is thus an uninterrupted chain of rhythmic breaths, in and out, until with his last breath man 'expires', i.e., 'breathes out' and closes the final link in the chain.

Our body carries within itself the four basic elements of the ancients, and our food, too, is correspondingly diversified. Our forefathers expressed it thus: 'We were made of *earth*, so we eat solid food; we were kneaded with water and hence drink liquids; the mind gives sense to the lifeless mass, therefore we breathe *air;* and with divine *fire* the spirit animates the composite whole so that it becomes man. 'While we can survive for weeks without solid foods and several days without water, life without air is only possible for a few minutes. This shows

48

that the connection between life and breath is the closest and that breathing is therefore the most important biological function of the organism. Every other activity of the body is closely connected with breathing. Breathing is of capital importance for our state of health, our emotional outlook and even for our longevity.

According to Indian philosophy, an individual is only given a certain number of breaths for each incarnation. One who breathes hurriedly and hastily dies sooner because he cannot take more breaths than the number prescribed. On the other hand, one who lives quietly and breathes slowly, husbands his store of health and will have a long life on earth. The people of the East do not get excited easily, because they—wisely enough —want to use their earthly life for spiritual progress. They shake their heads when they watch their brethren in the Occident shorten the divine gift of life by feverish activity and a resulting rapid, shallow breathing.

Civilized man does not know how to breathe! Our unnatural living conditions in modern city apartments and our cramped working conditions in factories and offices have resulted in our forgetting the rhythm of primitive breathing. Our stunted emotional life, and vacillation between passion and fear constrict our throats, and in the truest sense of the word, we do not dare to breathe deeply. *The way in which children in this twentieth century breathe is scarcely enough for the merest vegetating.* Their gasping is scarcely sufficient to keep them alive. How quickly this would change if people understood the ancient truth: *Only by the conscious regulation of our breathing can we achieve the resistance which assures us a long life free of sickness.*

Neglectful and haphazard breathing shortens our years, reduces our vital force and makes us susceptible to the mildest of all illnesses—the common cold.

Primitive man who lived under natural conditions did not need to be taught how to breathe. Hunting, fishing, struggle against the elements, the inclemencies of the weather, and constant movement in open air provided abundant natural exercise and made him instinctively a good breather. If we lived a normal, natural life, our bodies and our lungs would also show

49

the same reaction to outside influences as was the case with primitive man or African natives.

It will suffice to mention one example out of many thousands. In the summer time, when we escape from the heat and take refuge in cold water or when we are surprised by a sudden shower during an outing, what is our body's first reaction to the external stimulus? Instinctively, even against our will, we take a deep breath! Or let us stand under the shower early in the morning! The water need not even be cold; lukewarm will do. What happens? Immediately our chest, as if following a primitive command, rises and falls as long as the external stimulus on our skin continues. The wise men of India recognized, thousands of years before modern medical science was even dreamed of, that the skin is a second lung, for without skin breathing there can be no life. *Every external stimulus which reaches our skin—cold, heat, mechanical contact, etc.— automatically affects the rhythm of our lung breathing.*

Deep breathing, which is indispensable from the point of view of health and vital energy, is thus forced upon us numerous times each day by 'Mother Nature'. Unfortunately, however, *for civilized man who has cut himself off from natural living, there is only one way for nature to make him think of his health—through sickness.* Civilized man closes the pores of his skin with heavy and unnecessary clothing, thus completely inhibiting a more powerful activity of the skin and—in conjunction with the lungs —the beneficial effect of external stimuli on the vegetative nervous system.

After the Occidental has deafened himself for all time to the admonitions of wise nature in regard to health, strength, and longevity, there is only one way left for him directly to influence his lungs—through sports. What is the situation in the Occident in regard to sport and health? The twentieth century city dweller is compelled to live an unnatural cooped-up life. Even when he leaves his desk in the evening, tired out from his day's work, and takes the bus or the 'suburban' to get home sooner, he has neither time nor inclination for exercise. Very possibly this same person while living close to nature during childhood or youth, ran, swam or played in one of his school's teams. He may even have been quite a success at one sport or another. During adult life, however, only very few Europeans and Americans practise sports systematically. In the very years when we should be most concerned with keeping our health and maintaining the elasticity of our muscles, ninety per cent of us are not masters of our health but slaves of our professions.

Our way of living that involves so much sitting, or long hours of standing—and consequently flat feet—or bending over a desk has caused modern man to forget how to sit, walk, stand and breathe. The result is a sunken chest, narrow shoulders, asthma, circulatory disorders, arterio-sclerosis, diabetes, and tuberculosis—whereas a single generation of proper breathing would suffice to regenerate the race! An old Indian proverb says: 'It is not the same whether all the corners of a room are swept clean, or only the middle.' However, the fact that modern man is content with merely 'sweeping out the middle of his lungs' is evident from the following example.

According to occidental medical science, a person sitting quietly at work generally breathes fifteen times per minute. Nevertheless, at each breath, only about *half a quart of air is inhaled*. With somewhat deeper breathing, the amount of air passing into and out of the lungs is about $1\frac{1}{2}$ *quarts*, and a *further* $1\frac{1}{2}$ *quarts* of 'reserve air' passes through the lungs when we increase our breathing some more. The lungs of an adult thus have about $3\frac{1}{2}$ quarts of 'live volume' which is indicated by the fact that the lungs of corpses have been proved to contain $1\frac{1}{2}$ *quarts* of 'left-over air'. What does all this mean? No more and no less than that an Occidental living a sedentary life utilizes only one tenth of the five quart capacity of his lungs.

During a slow stroll, this amount is increased to two and a half times the capacity of the lungs; during mountain climbing, it jumps to ten times the lung capacity, and in swimming, to twenty times.

The wise men of India and the Orient recognized thousands of years ago the amazing results of regulating the breathing for maintaining health and warding off diseases. That is why they practically made religious ceremonies out of deep breathing exercises combined with contemplative physical postures. They intended that such exercises should be practised diligently by the masses every day.

51

In our times, however, Hatha Yoga in India has already been removed from the magic realm of mysticism. With the financial aid of Sir Natawarsinhaji Bahadur Maharaja and Rana Sahib of Porbandar, a research laboratory has been established in the city of Lonavla, in Poona. In this laboratory the physical exercises of Yoga are tested with the most up-to-date scientific instruments, and the amazing results are confirmed by medical observation. Before we take up the question of what the Yoga breathing method actually is, we should like to discuss why proper breathing is so exceedingly important, and thus we come to the question:

V

———————

What is Prana?

MANY thousands of years ago the enlightened wise men of the East taught that every force and all energy active in the universe had some inner cause, a core, a germ—a primaeval condition out of which all life, every movement and all activity arose. This potential force in its original condition is called 'prana'. Before the beginning of the creative cycle, prana lies dormant in the absolute as the spirit or the idea of all forces.

This immediately calls to mind the commencement of the Gospel according to St. John: 'In the beginning was the Word, and the Word was with God, and the Word was God. The same was in the beginning with God. All things were made by him; and without him was not any thing made that was made. In him was life; and the life was the light of men.' The 'Word' of the Bible and the 'prana' of the Oriental is one and the same concept. Only the name is different.

The beginning of creation means that prana 'awakens', begins to act, and that all kinds of forces come from it. Likewise all matter develops out of an original substance. In its latent condition, this original substance is the idea or the spirit of substance. Oriental philosophy calls this 'akasha'. In the commencement of creation, prana begins to act on akasha, shaping and moulding, and there are produced the countless varieties of force and substance. In every form of life prana is present as a living force which serves to help the all-animating Overself to unfold on the material plane.

Every force is based on prana; the force of gravity, attraction, repulsion, electricity, radio-activity—without prana there is no life, for prana is the soul of all force and all energy. This prime principle is to be found everywhere in the world. It is in the air, but is not air; it is in food, but is not food; it is the strength in the vitamin; it is also contained in water, but is not identical with the chemical constituents of water; these are merely carriers of prana.

The air is filled with free prana, and the human organism can most easily absorb prana from fresh air through the process of breathing. In breathing normally we take in normal amounts of prana. Through deep breathing our intake is increased, and *through controlled Yoga breathing we are able to store up a substantial quantity of reserve prana in our brain and nerve centres* to be used in case of necessity. There are people who, when suddenly thrown out of their every-day routine through some unusually great physical or mental emergency, do not collapse under the unaccustomed burden, but are able to perform astonishing feats of endurance. Such people unconsciously possess the ability to store up reserve prana. They are said to possess 'great vitality'. This 'vitality' is nothing else but reserve prana.

Concerning the prana theory it may suffice to state that it is not contradictory to the view held by occidental natural science. Western scientists also believe that the entire universe is filled with 'ether'. What this ether—which actually corresponds to prana—consists of, however, is a question to which occidental science fails to give a satisfactory answer. Let us merely think of the cosmic rays, these emanations which are constantly reaching our earth from distances many light years away. In the invigorating brilliance of these infinitely short wave-length radiations we live and flourish like a green twig in the spring sunshine.

Our body which consists of myriads of molecules and atoms is also permeated by ether—prana. Wherever there is life or motion in the universe, from the lowest animals on up to the greatest solar systems, without prana all would be only inanimate matter. This wonderful principle of life is the mother and the origin of all mental, chemical and physical force. According to the Vedanta philosophy, prana is the innermost intelligence of the 'natural forces' and their forms of manifestations. Invisible, immeasurable and indestructible—like all energy—yet not identical with the force of molecular attraction, but much finer than this, prana is the cosmic force of life, and its influence is to be found in every vibration on earth. The little seed germinates in the spring; life begins in the molecules of the cell, in the protoplasm. However, the living cell not only manifests vitality, but also intelligence. According to Yoga, there is an elective affinity between prana and mind, a relationship akin to that existing between horse and rider. The animal organism is, in fact, nothing other than the manifested form and mechanism of mental force. The mind which wants to manifest itself on the material plane, develops the appropriate organs with the aid of prana and constructs a living material body corresponding to its purpose on earth. Prana is thus the vital vibration which fills the universe.

Of all the universal prana which fills the universe, the prana active in our mind, brain and body is the nearest to us. We only attain harmony with the ocean of prana throughout the universe when we are able to guide the wave of prana that animates our material body, making it subservient to our will. The absolute master and controlling force of prana is thought! Thought is the key with which we can open or lock the door of LIFE in front of us. If we have made ourselves sick through creating wrong thoughts, then we can get well again with intentionally created right thoughts. (See also the chapter: 'The Constructive Power of Consciousness'.)

The seemingly marvellous results of hypnotism become comprehensible if we understand the connection between thought and prana. The hypnotist *collects and controls* the prana in the medium with the air of spoken thoughts. Indian Yogis, however, make no use of this power they have; for they believe that *no one has the right to interfere with the self and freedom of action of another person*. They likewise do not use hypnotism for healing purposes, because the results are not permanent. If the person who has been healed by another's intervention continues to make the same mental mistake as before, and if he continues to think wrong thoughts, the disease reappears with renewed vigour. Hatha Yogis teach their pupils how to *control and store up prana themselves*—that is, they teach them autosuggestion—so that they will not be dependent on the help of others, but on the contrary, resistant to all outside influences.

The purpose of Yoga is to liberate and develop the values in every human being, in order to activate the mighty mental and spiritual treasures which lie dormant in each individual—suppressed through wrong education, false opinions, pusillanimity, lack of self confidence, inhibitions and fears. Thus through Yoga, every one can unburden his soul and attain confidence in himself, and—as a direct consequence—his physical health. True healing can only take place when health is not left to outside influences or mere medication; the healing powers must be awakened *within the patient himself*!

If we want to be well, we must first of all *believe* in our health. If we believe in a thing, we will also fight for it! Let us imagine ourselves as absolutely healthy! The negative individual with his ailing mind is always a hypochondriac and does just the opposite. He continually imagines and believes himself to be sick. No wonder that irregularities of a thousand kinds appear until finally he is really sick. Let us fight for our health! Let us take the trouble to do something for it! Just as we take time to wash every day, we should take a little time, ten minutes or a half an hour, to give our body what it absolutely needs to carry on its hard work. Along with our daily *bread*, let us give our body the daily *strength* to digest this bread.

This strength is prana!

The most obvious manifestation of prana in the human body is the fact that it forces us to breathe. The result of this is the movement of our lungs. If we wish to get better acquainted with prana and learn consciously to store up more prana in our nerve centres, our first task is to control the movements of our lungs, that is, our breathing. This means that we cease to breathe haphazardly, irregularly, and unconsciously, and that we learn to take each breath consciously, with concentration of thought, leading the absorbed prana into the nerve centres that serve as storage areas. The conscious practice of controlling prana through concentration and regulated breathing is called pranayama. Pranayama is the most important basis of the system of Hatha Yoga. Prana is the fuel of the lung and the entire human body. If, through injury or a disease resulting from unnatural living, the body becomes incapable of absorbing prana, the powerful life current is turned off just as the current of a trans-

56

mitter ceases to flow through a damaged wireless set. It is still present in the universe, but it can no longer manifest itself. From the foregoing we are quite justified in stating, even in European terms, that without prana—whether we wish to call it ether, cosmic radiation or some other name—there could be no life on earth.

We can most easily curb disease and likewise increase and maintain our life force if we give our organism more and fresher prana. Hatha Yoga and the pranayama it teaches must not be considered in the occident as a theory laden with oriental hocus-pocus. Pranayama is quite deserving of serious attention by western physicians.

VI

_____

Complete Breathing

THE first and most important rule for right breathing is: Breathe through the nose! It is astonishing that civilized man who spends half his life acquiring an education, has not yet learned this most elementary rule of health. If we but knew what dangers we can escape through breathing through the nose, we would not be so negligent. According to my own observation, the majority of people in the Occident breathe through the mouth—especially in speaking. They also neglect to pay even the slightest attention to breathing through the nose while they are asleep. I am moved to pity at the sight of little children breathing through their mouths, while their otherwise intelligent and educated parents do not even make the slightest effort to break their children of this bad habit. The result is that the child's thyroid gland is stunted, and its mental development is retarded. The child is even in danger of feeble-mindedness. At the same time, its adenoids become enlarged and—in occidental practice—are then trimmed through an operation. With proper breathing all this would be unnecessary. The child does not breathe through the mouth because of enlarged adenoids, but rather the adenoids have become enlarged because of the mouth breathing. If we teach the child to breathe properly, parallel with appropriate Yoga exercises, the enlarged adenoids can be brought back to normal size.

The gateway to the air passages is the nose! Nature has equipped it with all necessary defence devices, so that neither impurities, nor excessively cold air, nor poisonous gases can enter the body. At the entrance of the nose, a little screen of hairs blocks the way for dust, tiny insects and other things that might injure the lungs. Then follows a long, winding passage-way lined with mucous membranes where overly cool air is warmed and dust particles, so fine as to have passed the hair screen, are precipitated. Such dust can easily be removed by vigorously expelling air through the nose—instantly ridding us of millions of bacilli. Then in the inner nose we have another team of gate-keepers. Glands fight off any bacilli which have penetrated so far and they are seconded by our olfactory organ, this remarkable instrument which immediately sounds the alarm whenever fermenting or putrifying substances menace our health with their poisonous gases.

The most important duty of our olfactory organ—a matter which is completely unknown in the Occident—is the *absorption of prana from the air*. The olfactory organ and the olfactory surface is not only a signal device for scents and odours, but also the inlet valve for prana. Should anyone doubt the truth of this statement, a single test should convince him. Everyone can make the experiment himself. When we are hiking in the high mountains or along the beach where prana is plentiful (in the Occident one says the air is rich in 'ozone'), we breathe deeply and immediately feel the great freshening 'lift' augmenting our strength. Now let us breathe in the same amount of air through the mouth, and the refreshing effect is lacking. The air absorbed through the mouth is flat and tasteless—it lacks the ozone-scent, the prana. And yet we have breathed the same air. When we have a bad cold and cannot breathe through the nose, how quickly we lose strength, how much we miss the quantity of prana normally absorbed through the nose! Many persons suffer weakness of the heart when they have a bad cold. The deficiency of prana is the reason.

In the mouth there is no organ for absorbing prana. Only the chemical substance in the air is absorbed. It is therefore obvious that if a person breathes through his mouth for a long period of time, he is bound to be seriously deficient in prana. He becomes weak, his glands function inadequately, vital processes are lowered, his whole body sinks into a negative state, and his resistance drops so low that he is defenceless against every kind of disease. Even worse, by breathing through the mouth, he by-passes the germ filter in his nose, thus putting himself completely at the mercy of infectious diseases whose pathogenic agents enter his lungs from the air.

The Nose Protects us from the Bacteria in the Air.

The mouth lacks defensive devices like those of the nose. The task of the mouth is partly to protect the body from other types of bacteria, but mainly to defend the oesophagus, to warn us, arrest and expel pips, fish bones and toxic substances of foul taste, so that these things do not reach the stomach. The job of filtering the air, however, belongs to the nose. To be sure, the mouth too is able to absorb the chemical components of the air. This wise precaution of nature, however, is only for our protection in the event that the openings of the nose are blocked as a result of sickness or accident, so that life can continue without interruption during the period of healing. The nose, too, is able partially to perform the task of the mouth; in case of emergency, a person can be fed through the nose. But a healthy person would never think of stuffing his food into his nose. Then why does he breathe through his mouth?

Every Organ Should Serve its True Purpose.

The basic requirement for the preservation of our health is to accustom each organ to perform its task perfectly. Let us breathe through our nose—always! This will give us supreme protection against infectious diseases. The abundant intake of prana through the nose will, with the help of the lungs, completely supply our body with energy. Primarily this will strengthen our heart which pumps blood and sends prana, via the blood-stream, into the tiniest blood vessels. Thus nose breathing has an effect on the activity of our brain. This also protects us against disease, as the resistance of mucous membranes and the glands is promoted by the additional supply of prana. This explains the case of countless patients suffering from general weaknesses; as soon as they get accustomed to breathing through the nose, they almost miraculously recover strength, get more enjoyment out of life, and are cured in no time from their chronic debility and fatigue.

If children were taught nose breathing in school, it would be possible to raise a new, stronger, and more intelligent generation!

The basis and the beginning of all breathing exercises is the so-called complete Yogi breathing. This consists of a synthesis

60

of three manners of breathing: 1. abdominal breathing, 2. middle breathing, and 3. upper breathing. In order to understand complete Yogi breathing, we must first understand its three parts.

Let us first consider the upper or shallow breathing which, in the Occident, is called clavicular breathing. About ninety per cent of all European women breathe in this way. We shall soon see why. In this type of breathing which raises only the ribs, the shoulders and the collar bone, only the upper part of the lung is used. As this is the smallest part, only a very small amount of air reaches the lungs. Since the diaphragm is raised the lung cannot expand downwards. The most elementary knowledge of anatomy is enough to convince every one that clavicular breathing consumes the most energy with the least results. *Most disorders of the vocal cords and the respiratory organs are the result of deficient breathing.* This is the easiest way to catch cold or fall into the habit of breathing through the mouth.

The fact that most women unconsciously practise shallow breathing—without having the faintest idea they are doing so as long as they live—is not due to any anatomical difference between the thorax of a man and that of a woman. The true cause is that, in order to keep slender, women force themselves into corsets, girdles and garter belts which have a pernicious effect, as they impede abdominal breathing, hinder the circulation of blood and the humours, and hamper the functioning of the abdominal organs. The condition is aggravated by the unnatural way in which women live and the fact that women's activities—sewing, handwork, bridge, etc., not to mention typewriting—require them to work in a hunched-over posture. If we bend over a typewriter or our handwork for one or two hours we are completely unable to take in air in any other way than upper breathing. The lower ribs are pressed in an acute angle over the diaphragm and keep the air from flowing downward.

But improper breathing is not confined to women. Among singers, the clergy, lawyers, and speakers there are very many whose breathing is quite faulty. The cause is not only our civilized way of living itself, but also the biological law by which every modern male city-dweller who has an unnatural way of

61

living, immediately relapses into shallow breathing as soon as his profession makes great demands on his lungs.

After all the foregoing, if any one still has the slightest doubt about the damaging effect and the reprehensibleness of shallow breathing, I can give him the following advice. Standing upright at attention with hands rigidly at the sides, lift the shoulders a little and breath deeply. Then throw back the head and drop the shoulders, and immediately you see that *you can breathe in still more*—at least as much more as before.

Second test. Let us sit at our desk leaning over forward a bit, just as we do while working. Our breathing again will be shallow, as our shoulders are in an unnaturally high position.

This explains why more and more men living in large cities are lapsing from lower to upper breathing.

Now let us consider the second unnatural occidental way of breathing, so-called middle—or as European doctors name it—inter-costal breathing. Most people who do not lead sedentary lives breathe like this. This middle breathing is one degree better than upper breathing, for it involves at least a little bit of abdominal breathing, and, instead of the upper lung, the middle lung is filled with air. This is the way most men breathe when they stand erect or sit—especially in a room with bad air, at the cinema, in the theatre or in a room where the windows are closed. Nature is instinctively reluctant to let us breathe deeply of stale air, and we resort to hasty inter-costal breathing. Let us observe ourselves the next time we are at the cinema.

Nature never completely abandons deep breathing. Even the person who leads the most unnatural city life often takes a deep breath spasmodically and convulsively, especially when he is in good air. *This is a desperate reflex movement, similar to yawning, made by the air-starved, stunted occidental lung.*

Abdominal breathing is also called deep breathing or diaphragmal breathing. Most men breathe this way when lying down or resting. This is the type of breathing advocated by European and American health lecturers, whereas actually it is only *part* of complete Yogi breathing. This abdominal breathing is used by strong Americans and Europeans who have a good physique and a healthy vocation. Most men can breathe abdominally because they do not wear corsets, girdles or similar constricting

62

garments, and their lungs are thus less abused by the conventions of civilized life. It should be emphasized, however, that the purest form of abdominal breathing is only found among strong, healthy men, soldiers, athletes, farmers and mountain shepherds.

The reason why this manner of breathing is called abdominal or diaphragmal breathing is immediately clear when we consider the location of the diaphragm. In other ways also the diaphragm plays an important role in the pranayama of the Yogis, and it will be useful to get acquainted with its function. The diaphragm is a strong partition of muscles separating the chest and the abdomen. At rest, it arches upward towards the thoracic cavity. When it is functioning, it flattens out more and more, thus pressing the abdominal organs downward and arching the abdomen outwards.

In shallow breathing, the upper part of the lung fills up with air; in middle breathing, only the middle and a bit of the upper part; and in deep breathing, the entire lower and middle parts. Hence, this kind of breathing is better than the two forms just discussed.

From the foregoing it is obvious that the most perfect method of breathing is that which fills the lower, middle and upper part of the lungs in the same way, thus supplying the organism with the maximum amount of oxygen and prana. This method is the ancient Yoga breathing which we shall describe in further detail.

The complete and perfect Yoga breathing contains all the advantages of abdominal, middle, and upper breathing, and none of their disadvantages. It brings the entire respiratory system—every cell and every muscle—into action. The thoracic cavity can at last expand to its normal, natural volume, and the performance of the lungs can even be increased through the vigorous use of the costal or rib muscles. The diaphragm, too, functions regularly and provides a surprisingly beneficial biological effect through gently massaging the abdominal organs. This will be discussed more fully in a later chapter.

The complete Yogi breathing is the simplest and most indispensable basis of all Yogi breathing. It scarcely need be emphasised that we must begin gradually and avoid over-exerting ourselves at the start. Too much of anything is very dangerous to health, and this is true of the erratic and disordered practice of pranayama

The reader will recall my own example after I had read my first book on Hatha Yoga and then in a surge of enthusiasm did Yoga exercises helter-skelter for hours at a time. *'Let the pupil go his way with patience'*, says an Indian proverb, *'or else his foundation and his too hastily constructed building will crumble in ruins about him'*.

The basic exercise for complete Yogi breathing is as follows:

Standing erect in normal, restful posture (Figure 1), we exhale vigorously and then breathe in, our inhalation being composed of the following three interconnected phases: 1. *By moving the diaphragm, we slowly push the abdomen outwards.* That is, we arch out the abdomen without consciously breathing in. In so doing, *we make the surprising discovery that merely expanding our abdomen has caused air to flow into the lower part of our lungs.* It is a good idea—at least in the beginning—to put the palms of both hands on the abdomen in order to note its movement. Men will find that this first phase of Yogi breathing, lower or abdominal breathing, is not difficult; for every healthy man is an abdominal breather. I was amazed, however, to find that at least half of the European women who neither practise sports nor take exercise are completely unable to breathe with the abdomen (diaphragm). I implore my feminine readers not to proceed further until, with all their concentration and will power, they have learnt how to perform the abdominal breathing without effort or special difficulty. Among my pupils in India and in Europe I have found that of the fifty per cent of the women who only know how to breathe with the upper part of their lungs and are thus unable to perform abdominal breathing at the first attempt, nearly all—almost without exception—are suffering from digestive difficulties, stomach trouble, chronic constipation, or various gynaecological disorders. Their abdomen is completely lifeless, as 'inanimate' as if it were a foreign object instead of part of their own body.

In the second phase of this breathing, we spread our lower ribs and the middle part of our thorax, so that little by little *the air streams into our middle lungs.* This phase corresponds to middle breathing.

The third rhythm in the inhalation is the full arching-out of the chest. With this motion we draw in as much air as we can get

64

into our expanded lung. In this last phase, we draw in our abdomen so it can act as a support for the lungs and at the same time, the upper lobes of the lungs can fill up full of air. The last rhythm is thus a completely performed upper breathing.

At first glance it seems as if Yogi breathing consisted of three rhythms of movement. However, this is only theoretically so, for in performing this breathing we must glide from one movement into the next, without a break or interruption. Seen from the side of the body, the perfect Yogi breathing appears to be a single, slow wave-like movement from the abdomen upwards. With a little practice, we are able to draw in the air evenly, with a smooth transition as we pass from one phase to the other.

Now we begin exhaling slowly through the nose so that we force the air out in the same sequence in which it was admitted. First we draw in the outer wall of the abdomen thus pressing the lower ribs together, and finally we lower the collar bone and the shoulders. In exhaling we press the abdominal and rib muscles together to such a degree that as little air as possible remains behind. Naturally we must not be violent about it.

A half hour before each of the three main meals we practise this simplest form of pranayama, at least one minute on the first day. Each day for the next five days we increase the dose by one minute. Not until then can we start on the other variations of Yogi breathing, for the above described basic exercise is the ABC for further progress.

Let us examine the effect of perfect Yogi breathing—the advantages of lower, middle and upper breathing, perfectly combined—as recorded in the teachings of the wise men of India and the experimental results attained by the Research Laboratory for Indian Yoga at Lonavla.

According to Yoga, the daily exercise of the simplest form of pranayama makes one almost immune to tuberculosis and other pulmonary disorders. One who systematically practises Yogi breathing exercises will neither get colds nor bronchial catarrh. For what, after all, is tuberculosis?—A *decrease in vitality* resulting from insufficient air, i.e., improper breathing. The reduced vital force lowers the resistance of the organism and provides a favourable culture medium for infectious germs.

65

Good, healthy lung tissues *resist* the bacteria. We can only achieve healthy lungs through *using* them properly.

Tubercular persons are generally narrow-chested. In most cases, this imperfect development comes from a wrong mental attitude. People with inferiority and fear complexes draw their shoulders forward and upward and thus press their thorax together. One can often notice this bad habit among children. The result is that the compressed lungs can scarcely breathe. As the proper expansion of the thorax is lacking, the lungs cannot develop properly. The supply of air is inadequate. This causes a constant shortage of oxygen and prana in the blood. Now we know that a weakened body which has got into a negative condition is a hotbed for tuberculosis bacilli. In addition we must remember the following: People who suffer from inferiority complexes are unhappy and generally seek an escape in sex. It is well known that children who have been repressed by their brothers and sisters and who feel that they are not sufficiently loved by their parents, resort to the dangerous practice of masturbation. However, excessive sexuality over-excites the entire glandular system including the hilar lymph node; the lungs develop catarrh and the tuberculosis bacilli have an open road. We see what a pernicious chain reaction can be set off by a negative mental attitude and inadequate breathing.

In many cases complete healing can be achieved in a short time if the patient breaks his habit of shallow breathing and begins to breathe deeply and thoroughly. Deep breathing also changes his mental attitude,—for how can a person who has a broad, well expanded chest and who breathes slowly and deeply, be fearful?

The well-aired lungs transmit more oxygen and prana to the body, the circulation is more vigorous, the whole body is relieved, breathes deeply, gets stronger, the sickness disappears.

Tuberculosis bacilli cannot thrive in thoroughly aired lungs charged with healthy blood. (See Chapter III).

According to Yoga teachings, the quality of the blood depends for the most part on the oxygen and prana absorbed in the lungs. If it contains only little prana and oxygen, its quality is inferior. Then it fills up with wastes and toxins which are improperly eliminated, and the whole body is burdened with impurities. Not only the organism but each individual organ is affected by the poor quality of the blood. The stomach and the organs of digestion generally suffer greatly as a result of inadequate breathing. The food withdraws oxygen from the blood, since before digestion and assimilation begin, a process of oxidation is necessary. However, if the assimilation is not normal, the organism does not get enough nourishment, physical strength declines, and vitality diminishes.

All of these evils can be prevented by right breathing. Not only the lungs and stomach are affected by improper breathing, but the entire nervous system, the brain, the spine, the nervous centres—even the nerves themselves—as they do not get enough prana and fresh oxygen.

The diaphragm which functions naturally during Yoga breathing puts a mild pressure on the liver, the stomach and the stomach organs, and this pressure, as a result of the rhythm of the lung breathing, is transformed into a gentle massage which promotes a natural functioning of the internal organs. As a result, every single breath has an effect on the abdominal organs, stimulating the blood circulation in these organs and increasing the metabolism. This beneficial inner massage is lacking when we merely are breathing with the upper or middle lung.

The enthusiastic pioneers of occidental physical education systems should not forget *that exercising external muscles is not everything. The inner organs also need exercise.* Nature provided for this through right breathing. Gymnastics, wrestling, fencing and similar sports provide more favourable conditions for the internal organs than they could get in a flabby organism, but without breathing exercises, sports can never have as favourable an effect on the organism as the natural massage of rhythmic pranayama.

At this point someone might ask why deep breathing is so important in life. Why should we do breathing exercises when we can get the same effect through sports? When we run, fence, row or play tennis, our lungs function to their full extent; we are automatically forced to take deep breaths and thus, indirectly, we achieve the beneficial effects of Yogi breathing!

This is not true, however. During vigorous sports, the lungs actually do work to their full capacity, *but unsystematically, with spasmodic jerky movements and the increased oxygen intake is immediately consumed as a result of the constant loss of energy.* Without rhythm there is no life. From the vibrations of the atoms on up to the sunrise or the beating of the heart, everything in this world is dominated by rhythm. This explains why the continual rhythmic exercising of Yoga breathing either in restful exercises or exercises involving only little bodily movement has an incomparably greater and more beneficial effect on all our organs than indulging in sports just for the sport's sake.

It must be added that western sports are dynamic, active, whereas the bodily exercises of Hatha Yoga are passive. *In active sports we expend our strength and then have to lie down to rest.* In the passivity of Yoga exercises, however, *we collect a gigantic amount of energy which we store up within us.* It is like building a dam across a river. The force is stored up, and this gives us an immense reserve of power.

With Hatha Yoga exercises we build, in our passivity, a dam across the river of life and store up the disciplined forces. Thus, no matter how tired we are when we come from work, we can easily do passive Hatha Yoga exercises, as they cause no further fatigue. On the contrary, after doing them we are remarkably refreshed. Anyone who has ever tried them knows!——

The miraculous effect of *retained breathing can also be partly explained in that way.* The reader will notice that in doing the pranayama breathing exercises described in the Practical Part of this book, the Indians always *combine them with the retention of the breath over shorter or longer periods. This is actually breathing control which has a most astonishing biological effect on the organism.* As a child, probably everyone, out of curiosity or 'just for fun', has tried to hold his breath, perhaps in competition with other youngsters to see who could hold out longest. As an adult, however, the occidental is instinctively afraid of such a thing, being fully convinced that such 'senseless and and unnecessary experiments' could only harm him. Who knows, perhaps his lung might burst a blood vessel, or he might have a stroke because of not getting any more air. How childish this idea really is! We need only think of primitive man or the wild tribes living in God's free out of doors.

Disregarding for a moment the natural skin breathing mentioned above, in which every external stimulus causes the lung to react involuntarily with a deep inhalation and convulsive jerky retention of the breath, let us consider the sportsman or the person performing hard physical exercises. During these exercises, he cannot breathe continuously, even if his thorax rises and falls violently as a result of his muscular work. During vigorous physical activity, in order for the organism to have correspondingly more time for absorbing and distributing the additional oxygen and prana energy, nature herself makes the body breathe intermittently, even during its great exertions and heavy consumption of energy.

If we watch a javelin thrower, a discus thrower, a swordsman or tennis player, we can see how just before the supreme exertion of his decisive movement, the athlete holds his breath and often makes a whole series of movements before exhaling. The greater the muscular work or the power he is required to exert, the deeper will be his inhalation preceding it and the longer he will hold his breath. In a hundred yard dash, the runner scarcely takes a single breath as he approaches the finish. Among long distance runners it is a recognized rule that only the one who knows how to 'save his breath' can hope for success. The Yogis made this discovery thousands of years ago and recognized the fact that pranayama practised in connection with retention of breath, stores up large quantities of prana and is therefore of extraordinary beneficial effect, not only for the organs of breathing and digestion, but also for the blood and the entire nervous system. How much more prana is stored up in the organism as a result of long exercises performed in a resting condition or with very moderate physical movement, than when the body is performing heavy work and the additional energy is immediately consumed! In simple Yogi breathing exercises, these forces not only strengthen and refresh the body as in the case of sports, but also have a therapeutic effect on the organism.— Breath control, however, has a remarkable effect, not only because we consciously economize on oxygen and prana, but also because some of these breathing exercises establish order and equilibrium among the positive and negative currents which animate our body.

Breathing itself is actually an alternation between positive and negative conditions. In inhaling we are in a negative condition— we are receiving, drawing in the life-giving element. While exhaling we are positive—we distribute the power we have taken in to all parts of our body; we are giving, radiating. One who thinks logically will already realize that if we consciously control the regularity of our breathing, this in itself sets up an equilibrium between the positive and negative energies. *In holding his breath, a person is forced—at least for a time—to focus his consciousness in the centre of his SELF and to unite both energies.* As a result he achieves a condition of complete equilibrium, both mentally and physically. It is the same as if I were to stop an oscillating balance at the very moment when the pointer is at the centre, that is, when the balance is in complete equilibrium. When I take a sick person who has got out of equilibrium and, in a similar manner, bring him back to equilibrium, his healing is greatly aided. The alternating breathing exercises—such as 'Bhastrika' for example, that is, alternating breathing through the right and the left nostril—force the person to an even greater extent to establish equilibrium between the positive and negative forces in his body. In this way the body maintains its health. However, if it is already diseased as a result of the improper distribution of forces, it is brought back to equilibrium again and healed. This is the whole secret of the pranayama method.

By holding the condition of equilibrium—that is, by retaining our breath, we thoroughly clean all the little air sacks in the lungs and stimulate them to increased activity. In this way the stagnating impurities and toxins in the blood are vigorously expelled. The retained breath has somewhat the same effect on the lungs and the blood as a laxative on the organs of digestion. For this reason those who regularly practise Yogi breathing never suffer from disorders of the lungs, stomach, liver, gall or heart, nor do such persons include any asthmatics or sclerotics.

From the foregoing, it is clear, that not only from the oriental viewpoint, but also from that of occidental biology and medicine it is vitally important for every man, every woman, and every child to practise pranayama daily, if they wish to maintain their health and vital strength. The matter is so simple that the great masses do not even take it seriously, preferring to spend fortunes for complicated cures and medicaments. While health is knocking at their very door, they refuse to open it. *They commit the heinous sin of rebelling against recognized truth.*

70

VII

— — — — —

Swimming:
FOR PERFECT BREATH REGULATION

SWIMMING is the only sport whose beginnings are lost in the mists of prehistoric times and which, among all the ancient and modern types of physical pastimes is still considered *the most natural and perfect exercise even today*. There is not one other sport which has such beneficial effects on the health. We shall soon see why.

First of all, swimming is a natural exercise, not an artificial one. Secondly, even today it is the *only sport in the world which, because of the perfectly rhythmic movements required, forces us to breathe deeply in the pranayama manner*.

Thanks to these characteristics, swimming when practised regularly and in moderation is extraordinarily beneficial to the health. In order for this effect to be perfect, however, we must adapt our entire breathing technique to pranayama. Those who practise Yogi breathing daily and also conscientiously practise the ancient asanas (physical postures) described in the Practical Part of this book, can reach the highest degree of health and vital force; they will never be sick and according to Hatha Yoga Pradipika 'the shadow of their life will lengthen as rays of the slowly setting sun'. Such Yogis have no further need for any special sport.

The fact that I am devoting special attention to swimming has, in addition to the foregoing, a further special reason. I know from experience that most persons who practise pranayama wish to achieve quick success with the breathing exercises and often do not have sufficient patience to practise diligently for at least two months in succession. Prematurely discontinued pranayama exercises, however, are of no permanent benefit. Another mistake of the occidental beginner is that, after his first burst of enthusiasm has passed, he neglects the exercises, because the concentrated breathing actually does fatigue his lungs in the first few days; or he tires of the exercises because they last too long. Even in other ways, too, one must have strong will power in order not to relapse into the habit of shallow breathing.

I have placed such a great emphasis on swimming, because it is the only basic exercise which forces everyone to control his breathing. One must hold his breath for a certain length of time if he does not want to swallow water. Thus the careless 'Yogi breather' and the sceptical beginner can be led with the aid of swimming, to breathe in a manner similar to that prescribed by pranayama. *And a person who continues at least for two months in succession to practise the simple Hatha Yoga swimming exercises achieves the same results as through pranayama!* Thus if rapid results are desired and the individual is not strong willed enough to follow exactly the breathing rules from the very beginning, let him swim for one or two months in the Yoga manner.

In Madras I had an English Hatha Yoga pupil, an overweight officeworker, nearly forty years of age, who constantly complained that she could not lose weight. While still in her teens, she had enjoyed sports, swimming, and rowing—but dropped them all when she married and moved to India. In India she had so much work that there was no time for any exercises except short walks. From then on she had tried everything she could think of—organo-therapeutic preparations and laxative herb teas, all kinds of sports, even boxing!—but all in vain. She could not lose a single pound. And whenever she did lose a bit, she gained it back again immediately. Even reducing cures and diets failed to bring the desired results. I tried pranayama exercises with her but her lungs and her will power were both so weak that after three full breathings she was breathless and ready to give up. She was likewise unable to hold her breath, a fact which indicated an extraordinarily small lung capacity.

After I saw that it was useless to prescribe breathing exercises which she would not do at home anyway, I resorted to the method my old teacher Mohan Singh had used for backward

72

pupils. I asked Mrs. Potter whether she could swim, for everything depended on that. She answered that in her younger years she had been a good swimmer, and although she still knew how, she did not see any hope in swimming, as she had already tried it once without success. Despite the fact that swimming is generally supposed to be reducing, her own experience with it had been negative.

That afternoon shortly after sundown we went to the seashore together. In Madras the thermometer hovers about 95° to 105°F all through the day; so people do not go to the beach until the evening hours when the blasting heat has given way to a comfortable, balmy warmth. I took Mrs. Potter to a secluded spot free of waves. On the other side of the breakwater the 'wave riders' of Madras were playing their games. With shrieks of pleasure, they ran out into the water up to their necks, waited for the next big wave, lay down upon it and let its crest drive them in to the shore with express train speed. My pupil was puffing pitiably. She was bathed in perspiration. When we reached the quiet water, our lesson in 'weight reducing' began.

'Now, Mrs. Potter', I said, 'just get into the water and show me how you swim'.

I did not have to ask her twice. While we were still in the car, she had shed her beach costume and ended the drive in her swimming suit. She splashed into the water like a seal as if boasting that despite her 160 pounds, she had not forgotten how to dive. She reached her goal while I looked on with admiration at the smooth regularity of her breast stroke.

'Now we'll get results!' I thought.

'Mr. Yesudian', she called out puffing and blowing, 'if you could prove Archimedes' law with your Yoga, I would gladly stand on my head all day!'

'What do you mean?' I asked, not understanding her.

'Well', she explained, 'the old boy claimed that a body immersed in water loses an amount of weight equivalent to that of the water it displaces . . . and I'm sorry to say I don't feel a single ounce lighter than I did on the shore'.

'Excellent!' I thought. 'Mrs. Potter certainly does have a good sense of humour, and she knows how to use it'. In doing any physical exercise, a happy frame of mind is worth its weight in gold.

'My dear lady,' I exclaimed, 'I guarantee that even if right now you are not losing the equivalent weight of the water you displace, in two months' time you will be at least twenty pounds lighter. Let's start in just as if you had no idea about swimming. You get through the water fast all right, but now remember you're *swimming for your health's sake. You want to reduce.* This can only be done with breath control—therapeutic swimming'.

Mrs. Potter was so surprised that she dived under water for a moment and then came up puffing and blowing again.

'Stop pulling my leg'! she retorted.

'Now just you watch, Mrs. Potter', I answered, as I went to her side in the lukewarm water. 'You must remember that taking off and putting on weight both depend on certain internal organs of secretion. If for any reason these organs are not in equilibrium, that is, if the secretions or the circulation of the blood has changed, the thyroid gland functions improperly and loses its capacity to regulate your weight. If you are too thin or unnaturally heavy, or if you suddenly gain or lose weight, this is the result of a disorder. Such conditions cannot be cured with so-called reducing or weight-building regimens, tea, arsenic or medicaments. The remedies offered by organo-therapy also only work for a short time. Your organism, Mrs. Potter, must be made healthy. That is the only way to restore the equilibrium. If you are over-weight you must get back to normal, and if you are under-weight, you gain just as much as you need. . . .'

'And you believe that swimming will cure me? A year ago I went swimming regularly. By the end of two months I had gained two pounds!'

'It is not swimming that will restore you to health', I answered, 'but the breathing exercises you unconsciously do while you are swimming. Since I cannot force you to practise pranayama exercises, I will prove to you through 'Yoga swimming' that you will lose a few pounds within a month. For people who lack the patience to practise pranayama, 'Yoga swimming' is the only sport that can restore the functioning of their organs to normal. A natural result of the perfectly restored equilibrium is that the

74

over-weight person slenderizes and the thin person gains. . . .'

'I'd like to see that!'

'Then let us begin, Mrs. Potter! For the present we shall stick to the breast stroke as the most natural kind of swimming. No one can be a perfect swimmer until he learns to economize on his breath. Endurance swimmers unconsciously practise 'Yoga swimming'. They breathe less frequently and blow the air out of their lungs while their face is still under water. And that is all there is to it. You see, it is not as hard as it seems! . . . While swimming breast stroke one cannot breathe haphazardly; one is forced to do it like this.—While making the first stroke with the arms, you take in a big breath of air through the nose and immediately plunge your face into the water just as racers do when swimming breast stroke. But don't be in such a hurry! The whole secret of Yoga is smooth, easy, rhythmic swimming without exertion . . . And so after taking your first breath you put your head in the water. In this way you are forced to hold your breath. . . . Fine, you've done that very well!'

'In all the time I've known how to swim I've never thought of that!' said Mrs. Potter, as she popped her head out of the water. 'I've always been far more concerned about my permanent wave. . . .'

'Yes, that is a bad habit of the ladies', I answered. 'So now while your face is in the water take two smooth easy strokes. When you put your hands in front of your chest for the second stroke, start slowly blowing the air out of your nose under the water so that by the end of the second stroke when you lift your head out of the water, the remainder of the air in your lungs just suffices for a single short blow to clear the last drops of water out of your nose. . . . At the same moment you quickly take a deep breath, put your head back into the water again and swim two more strokes in the same way. . . . With the help of this slow rhythmic swimming which is really nothing more than a perfect pranayama exercise in the water, you will come back to perfect health, provided you practise this daily and systematically. . . .'

Without doubt it was hard at the beginning. Mrs. Potter occasionally swallowed a mouthful of water and often had to stop for a minute to catch her breath. But regularly day after day she went out to the quiet bay and swam indefatigably according to my instructions.

Within a month and a half she had lost ten pounds, and by the end of the second month, eight pounds more. Thus I lost my bet by a mere two pounds. It is to Mrs. Potter's credit, however, that she did not blame me for this. On the contrary, from that day on she became one of my most eager pupils, coming to my classes early in order to practise pranayama. . . .

I recommend this method to everyone who can swim and lacks the patience to practise breathing exercises regularly. *After one or two months of daily Yoga swimming, his body will feel wonderfully well and healthy*. He will feel fresh and clean again and get more pleasure out of his work. If he neglects his swimming three or four days his lungs will crave their customary exercise as much as a smoker craves his cigarette. This is the moment when the pupil can gradually shift from swimming to regular pranayama practice in his room, or even better, out of doors. This wonderful system was used by my old master in my own case, because the daily practice of breathing control was so hard in the beginning. A number of my comrades were also very backward during their early training. Then Mohan Singh took us to the beach and taught us 'Yoga swimming'. After a month we could breathe better than the other pupils! . . . Swimming, practised simply, is the most perfect sport for breath regulation. In the summer time we should go to the sea shore or a lake or a river and swim in the Yoga method as often as we can spare the time. And let us not neglect this even in the winter! This ancient sport simultaneously strengthens our skin and, *as a result of the external stimulus, forces our lungs to perform such powerful work that no effort of will power is required. It is sufficient when the rhythm of our movements has been transmitted to our nerves*. One more rule should be noted in connection with swimming: On days when we go swimming, we should never stay more than half an hour, and we should omit our breathing exercises at home.

Breast stroke swimming with two strokes between each breath can be extended to several strokes after a few months. If we get tired, we must not stop but simply rest, floating on our back in the water and breathing deeply.

76

The most ancient and yet the most modern form of swimming is the crawl which the Hawaiian prince Kahanamoku introduced in the Occident at the beginning of this century. The crawl involves a perfect example of Yogi breathing. Powerful, deep breathing, kumbhaka (breath retention) during four strokes under the water, then blowing out the breath like a bellows through the nostrils, beginning while the face is still under the water. . . .

There is nothing new under the sun! If we study the rules of health, beginning with earliest recorded history on down to the most up-to-date hygiene, we are forced to admit that the precepts of our forefathers are still valid in many ways today and that this claim of ours sometimes surpasses our boldest dreams. In connection with swimming I must describe another unusual case which surprised me as much as it did Mr. John Kennedy, a salesman of the Ford Company in Calcutta. He was a young man, 5 feet 11 inches tall, and exceptionally thin. Every summer he spent a number of weeks with his relatives in Madras. I made his acquaintance at the beach. I noticed that in spite of his muscular though very thin physique, he spent hours on end in his tent and only went into the water after sundown for four or five minutes, then came right out again. That was all the exercise he took, despite the fact that he swam so excellently! One noticed that he felt completely at home in the water. He would surface dive, swim breast stroke, back stroke, crawl, and then rush out of the water as if something had bitten him.

When I asked the reason for his peculiar behaviour, I received the following surprising reply:

'You've hit my worst trouble', he said. 'In my youth I was a keen swimmer and there wasn't a day when I didn't spend some time in the Newark swimming pool. . . . But this race for speed, speed, speed! Do you know what life is like in the USA? Having to earn a living forced me to give up sports. For ten years I haven't had a bit of exercise. In hustling and rushing about I've lost so much weight I could weep every time I look in the mirror. I used to weigh 165 pounds but now I'm down to 132! No matter how much I eat, I don't gain a bit. . . .'

'Why don't you practise sports?' I asked amazed. 'You have time enough as I see from the fact that you spend several months here every year. For days I've watched you swim for only a moment or two and spend all the rest of your time in your tent. In the evening you scarcely swim three minutes and then bounce out of the water again!'

'That's just the trouble!' he exclaimed bitterly. 'My every fibre craves water but I don't dare swim as I'd like to, because I'm afraid I'll lose even more weight. They say swimming is the one thing in the world that takes off weight faster than a steam bath'.

This naive idea made me smile. I determined to take the matter in hand and explain my friend's mistake to him. This poor fellow spending day after day at the beach, yearning for water! It was really too bad; for swimming was just the thing to correct his condition. Cautiously I began to tell him about Yoga exercises and asked whether he had ever heard about prana-yama. He did not know what it was. When I explained it to him he smiled patronizingly. 'Do you think you can make me put on weight by *breathing*?' he echoed. 'Stop your kidding, fellow!'

Then I explained in detail the advantages of Yoga swimming and assured him he would put on weight if he practised half an hour daily according to my instructions. He refused to listen, sceptical like most people in the West. A month later he was still lying on the beach all day long, not going near the water until the evening, and then only for a moment like the Finns when they rush out of their steam baths and jump into cold water. In September the next year I saw John Kennedy at the Madras beach again. This time, much to my surprise, he was not lying in the sand so much but accompanying the sixteen and seventeen year old Indian boys during their wave riding. After a few weeks he became so skilful that he could go out into the water up to his mouth, then turn his back to the approaching wave, stretch out flat and let the wave drive him towards the shore as fast as an arrow. When he reached shallow water, he waded back to the noisy laughing group. I inquired about his new sport and he laughingly assured me he had found a way to enjoy himself in the water. In practising wave riding he was not forced to 'exert himself'. He did not need to swim a single stroke. He could walk leisurely into the water, wait until the next big wave came, then lie down upon it and be propelled to shore just like a board. 'Oh boy, it's great fun!' he called out enthusiastically. 'I've already gotten as good as a Kanak at Waikiki beach. This is a lot more fun than just lying around doing nothing in my tent. And I don't need to be afraid of losing weight because I don't have to swim a single stroke. . . .'

Shortly after this conversation I was called away from Madras for a month. When I returned, I went out to the beach on a hot, humid October day. Kennedy was enjoying himself with the youngsters. He had scarcely seen me when he began to gesticulate wildly and ran out of the water straight towards me. 'Man alive!' he called out breathlessly, 'a miracle has happened! I've been looking for you everywhere! . . . Yesterday I weighed myself in the hotel. . . . For two months I haven't bothered. . . . And now look—*I've gained eight pounds!* . . . Only I can't understand how in the world it's possible!'

This fired my keen interest. 'There is something definitely wrong', I said to myself. 'This man is not swimming; he is not making a single movement, simply letting the water carry him— and yet he is gaining weight . . .' Immediately I went with him to take part in the wave riding game, and by the very next day I had solved the riddle.

In expectation of the wave, the swimmer takes a deep breath and then lies down in the water with his face forward. As long as he is carried by the water he can only breathe at intervals. He takes a deep breath and is forced to retain it. This is repeated several times until he reaches shallow water. For at least thirty or forty seconds he is forced to retain his breath. John E. Kennedy was not swimming a single stroke and yet he was performing a perfect pranayama exercise, half an hour daily, day after day. When I explained the cause of the 'miraculous' gain in weight and the biological health controlling effect of breathing exercises, his opinion about Indian pranayama changed immediately.

'For breath is life', says an old Sanskrit proverb, 'and if you breathe well you will live long on earth.'

VIII

Civilized Appetite

THE Bible tells us that man was allowed to live in paradise as long as he had not eaten of the fruits of the tree of knowledge of good and evil. The very moment when he tasted of these fruits, however, God drove him from the Garden of Eden. What does this mean?

Man is a connecting link between spirit and matter. His highly developed brain enables him to manifest his divine SELF on the material plane. In order to do this he needs a material form, a cover: his body. His self is spiritual and creative, standing over the created form. His body, however, belongs to the material world ruled by the laws of nature. Animals are vehicles of nature, living in a closed circuit of natural forces, and therefore they cannot sin against nature. They manifest natural laws completely, automatically and directly. They are incapable of applying these laws at will, as they have no highly developed consciousness such as that of man. Thus they are always living in a state of paradise and cannot 'fall'.

Man, however, through his intelligence, has the possibility of getting acquainted with those laws. As long as he only learns and knows the laws of nature, the divine order is not disturbed, and he can continue to live happily in paradise. The tree of knowledge of good and evil stands before him—but he must not partake of its fruit; that is, he must not make *an end in itself* of his knowledge of natural laws. Nature reigns in our body through the two world-moving forces of the instinct of self preservation and that of the propagation of the species. The serpent in paradise, the great temptation, is just this very possibility of turning instinct into an end in itself. However, if man places his intelligence at the service of his instincts, he immediately 'falls' from his state of paradise and becomes unhappy. As long as he is not conscious of his spirituality, he actually uses his intelligence to make a source of pleasure out of the natural laws.

It is a natural law that the body must replenish its exhausted energies. It needs nourishment. Nature works in our body and when the organism needs food, the demand is signalled to us through a feeling which we call hunger. Inasmuch as hunger means that there is a deficiency, it is obviously our duty to overcome this shortage and eat. And since in our consciousness we experience the restoration of order through the operation of natural forces as pleasure, it is just as natural for us to take pleasure in satisfying our hunger. Recognizing this pleasure, man has made it an end in itself, a means of enjoyment. In other words, he has eaten of the fruits of his knowledge. He no longer takes food in order to maintain the efficiency of his body, but now considers eating to be a source of pleasure!

Intelligence stands over matter, over the body, but man has debased it and subordinated it to the body, making it into a servant, a slave of the physical. It was not enough for him to satisfy a healthy hunger; he went on to invent all kinds of stimulants in order to enjoy the pleasures of eating long after his body had no further needs! A supreme example of such a sinful attitude is found in the practice of the old Roman aristocrats who used a peacock feather to induce vomiting. With stomachs thus emptied, they could continue their feasting.

Man's palate now lost its natural reactions; it no longer reported to the brain that it needed nourishment to maintain the body. The overstimulated condition of the palate caused it to seek satisfactions—even when there was no necessity—and thus civilized appetite, man's constant craving for food and drink, was born.

Hunger is natural. It is nature's signal that the body needs food. Appetite is unnatural; for it only represents a wish to satisfy the overstimulated palate. And as this wish does not arise from a healthy need for food, we overburden our organs and make our bodies sick.

If we watch how people sin against their bodies, turning food and drink into a means to ruin their health, we need no longer wonder why there is so much unhappiness and disease on earth. Civilized man has become so accustomed to this unnatural way of eating and drinking that the abnormal seems normal to him, and he does not even notice how he is sinning against nature and his health. When we compare our way of eating with that of wild animals living according to nature's laws, we immediately recognize the terrifying difference between natural eating and drinking and 'civilized eating and drinking', which in reality is nothing but a constant craving for pleasure. Who has ever seen a thirsty animal that wanted to drink beer, wine or sweetened syrups diluted and charged with carbon dioxide?

From our own experience we know that after physical work and after perspiring freely, only pure water will completely quench our thirst—and at such times this is what we want to drink. But when we slake this real thirst, the water we drink has a delightful taste all its own, it has a long forgotten aroma. It is entirely different from what people seek when they merely want to enjoy something, when out of sheer habit they sit with friends in a café, tea room or bar, to chat and load their stomachs with some tasty stimulating liquids not in the least required by their body. Of all the beverages, beer, whisky, liqueur, cognac, and all the myriad kinds of aperitifs—none of them taste as good as pure fresh water after a few hours' work in the hot fields, a climb to a mountain rop, or some other healthy form of sport. What a difference there is between simple natural food eaten after physical exertion in order to satisfy a healthy hunger—and the over-refined, over-spiced 'good things' we take to gratify an over-stimulated civilized appetite.

Children and wild tribes living on a childlike plane of development still enjoy healthy natural hunger. Primitive races prepare their food very simply. They also eat fruit in a raw state.

Very early in life, however, children are spoiled by their environment. Parents and grand-parents want to win their young ones' love and give them sweets and chocolates. In this way, through falsely manifested affection, they spoil their children physically and mentally. On the physical side the child's healthy instinct is deadened; it accustoms itself to eating without being hungry, for the sake of enjoyment. Thus its craving for pleasure is awakened early in life. On the mental and spiritual side this arouses a selfish instinct in the child. At an early age it begins to take advantage of the love of its relatives by expecting gifts constantly and begging for them.

Irrational civilized man also spoils the animals living in contact with him. The unfortunate dogs, cats, birds and other creatures which are so unlucky as to become the pets of people who live unnaturally, lose their native instincts and develop a craving for tit-bits and dainties which they want to eat all day long without hunger, just as their masters do. And their masters, to please them, give them sweetmeats, which undermine their health and shorten their lives.

The whole question is excellently illustrated by the story about the old maid's dog.

An old maid took her pet lap dog to a veterinary. The dog was as fat as a sausage, and the good lady complained that he had lost his appetite. 'For a long time he has only eaten veal, cake, and cream', she said, 'but now he refuses to eat anything at all'. The veterinary consoled her: 'Just leave him here, I guarantee that in a fortnight he will be so completely cured that he will eat wild pears with great gusto'. Although scarcely believing, the lady did as the veterinary suggested and went home shaking her head. Two weeks later she returned to fetch her pet. When the veterinary brought him in she could scarcely recognize him. He was slender, vivacious, and agile. The doctor threw him two wild pears. Instantly the dog pounced upon them and devoured them voraciously. 'Doctor', exclaimed the lady, 'this is a miracle! How in the world have you done it?'—'Very simply', answered the doctor, 'those two pears are the first food he's had since the day you brought him here.'

The dog had recovered its natural hunger through a healthy fast. Its digestive organs had recovered from their over-burdened condition, its heart and blood circulation were relieved and strengthened through the slenderizing process, and its entire body had again become a manifestation of nature.

Civilized man's craving for pleasure not only shows up at meal times, but also in the train, at the theatre, at the concert, or the cinema. People are constantly picking and nibbling. We always have some chocolate in our pocket, and at every opportunity we stuff a piece in our mouth. How then can our digestion function properly?

This brings us to one of civilized man's greatest sins—the *temperature* of food and drink!

The refrigerator—a blessing when used properly—has been turned into a curse.

When used to keep perishable foods fresh, the refrigerator is a blessing. When misused to enable us to serve food and beverages ice cold, it is a curse. Ice cold food and beverages have an injurious effect as soon as they are in the mouth. The enamel of the teeth becomes cracked and loses its ability to fight off mouth bacteria. The result is tooth decay. The mucous membrane of the tongue is also affected. Without our noticing, its delicate sensitivity is impaired. The tongue has the task of recognizing the finest shades in taste so that we can guard ourselves against the entry of any kind of spoiled or poisonous food particles. A dull tongue, however, cannot perform this task perfectly! The mucous membranes of the throat and stomach are also affected; the gall bladder and the liver are seriously attacked. It is no wonder that such a frightfully high percentage of civilized people suffer from acid stomach, stomach ulcers, inflammation of the gall bladder, gall stones and liver and pancreas disorders. The most dangerous thing, however, is ice cold fruit. Fluids are more quickly warmed to body temperature than pieces of ice cold fruit, especially when they are not thoroughly chewed. Such pieces of badly masticated ice cold fruit lie for a long time in the stomach, not only cooling the mucous membranes of the stomach walls, but also all the organs in the vicinity.

Nearly the same can be said for hot foods and beverages. Whether the mucous membranes are attacked by cold or heat does not make a great difference. In any case experience shows that deviation from a healthy temperature in what we eat and drink paves the way for cancer of the throat, stomach, liver and pancreas.

Let us take the animals for example!—Have you ever seen a cat that drank milk ice cold or piping hot? In a number of languages a proverbial expression for hesitation is to 'go about doing something like a cat about hot mush'. Even when her unreasonable, irrational master gives her such a dish, the cat will wisely wait—no matter how hungry she may be—until the milk has cooled off or, if it is ice cold, until it has warmed a bit. Only then will she start to lap it up.

We must often look on with horror when we see well meaning but unknowing mothers give their little children lumps of ice to swallow whole. Such mothers are surprised when their children are attacked by violent vomiting and diarrhoea. Throughout their entire lives these children may suffer from chronic stomach and intestinal catarrh.

Yoga means that we live and act *with* nature and not *against* nature. We can only conquer nature when we not only know her laws, but also recognize and obey them.

The miller harnesses the gigantic power of the river to turn his mill wheel. However, he can only master and use this power if he builds his wheel according to the laws of hydraulics, that is, in conformity with natural power. We could give further examples of this.

Back to nature! Let us live, breathe, eat and drink naturally; then we will always be healthy. And if we have already harmed our bodies, the return to nature will help us even in seemingly hopeless cases.

During World War II, I was able to observe how after the siege of a large city, the people who had previously spent their entire day sitting in badly ventilated offices were now required to move away rubble, carry beams, pull carts and even build walls if they wanted to have a roof over their heads. Often they had to travel many miles on foot to get their food. The result was that even those who had been leading a life of suffering and misery due to digestive disorders, stomach ulcers, chronic stomach or intestinal catarrh, gall disorders or other diseases, and who had only been able to live by a strict diet, were suddenly able to eat the heaviest food—beans, yellow peas or cabbage—digesting such foods excellently. They were thoroughly cured of their ills! They lost their civilized appetite and recovered their natural hunger.

Let us not wait until destiny forces us to live naturally; let us begin *consciously* of our own free will to bring our vital functions back into their natural ways.

The Yogi conquers appetite and opens the way for the development of natural hunger. He only eats when he is actually hungry and chews each bite ten times as long as the occidental—until it is thoroughly insalivated, and he does not swallow it until it has been *chewed into a milky mush*. From the viewpoint of the prana current, this is extraordinarily important.

According to Yoga theory, all foods, especially raw green vegetables, fruit, milk, milk products and honey, are filled with prana which is absolutely necessary for the maintenance of life, energy and health. Just as the nose is designed to absorb prana in the air for the purposes of health, the mouth is the absorptive organ for prana in food. Every atom of our food contains an infinity of food prana, and the prana liberating through thorough mastication is absorbed by the organism. It penetrates blood, flesh, and bones in order to be stored up in our nervous centres so as to be available to the organism.

The occidental reader may rightly ask why the human being needs the food prana; why air prana is not sufficient? On this point Yoga states that just as electricity has various forms which affect the human body differently, prana in the air, food, and water—even though essentially the same—sets off different functions in the body. In respect to prana theory, the science of Yoga would fill volumes, but within the scope of this book I am unable to discuss it further. Let us therefore assume that food contains prana, as explained by the ancient Indian science, and that this prana is liberated by thorough mastication. In the West, in ancient times, there was also a great wise man Epicurus, who taught the same thing: 'You must get every bit of taste out of every bite if you want it to do any real good,' he taught. He knew that the true benefit of food was not only in its nutritional value but in this indwelling prime energy of prana. The taste lies in the prana.

Primitive man only obtained food at infrequent intervals, by the sweat of his brow, and in the face of great dangers. Because it came so seldom, he enjoyed and relished his food. This is also a commandment of nature; for according to the finding of western medical science, food must be thoroughly mixed with saliva for the stomach to be able to digest it. Occidental city dwellers are so predisposed to stomach disorders because they eat in a hurry and do not take sufficient time for chewing, so that their stomach is not able to cope with the inadequately masticated and hastily swallowed food. The mouth is the antechamber of the stomach, and nature has provided this tool with the most magnificent grinding equipment, the teeth. *If we do not use this grinding mechanism, how can we expect the stomach with its soft walls to cope with our food? It is forced to increase its chemical treatment and to produce stronger digestive juices and more stomach acid.* Hyperacidity of the stomach and the ulcers which result therefrom have their cause in our impatience and in our badly chewed food! And now a word about teeth. As a result of the great adaptability of nature, this organ, if not utilized in accordance with its design, degenerates and decays. In order to supply our teeth with an abundance of blood we must use them in accordance with nature's design. When we chew vigorously, our teeth obtain a generous flow of blood about their roots. There would be no brittle teeth if children were taught early in life to chew their food thoroughly. Among animals there are no decayed teeth and no stomach disorders, except among those animals which have been spoiled by the cooked and lifeless food of man and which are thus not forced to use their teeth according to nature's design.

Thorough mastication is very important for many reasons. In the Occident there are also apostles of this truth. In his famous book, Horace Fletcher tells us that every bite must be chewed thirty times before we swallow it and that it should be chewed partly on the right and partly on the left side. This will have an excellent effect on the digestion. The constant practice of this method will protect us from numerous stomach and intestinal disorders or heal us if we are already affected. Fletcher proclaims the correct method of chewing, without realizing that the abundant insalivation simultaneously promotes the absorption of prana.

For years I have been studying occidental medical works and the latest developments in therapeutics in order to see how much they differ from the principles of Hatha Yoga. I have been surprised to find that the latest discoveries of the most up-to-date European and American investigators—consciously or unconsciously—come ever closer to the rules of ancient Hatha

Yoga. In regard to food intake and mastication, the latest trends in modern nutrition coincide almost identically in all points with the ancient Indian teachings. From the Swiss Dr. Bircher-Benner to progressive physicians the world over, we find practically nothing but Yoga teachings in their published works.

When we have learned what proper mastication means, the question automatically arises: what diet should a Hatha Yoga pupil follow?

The authors of modern books on nutrition fill up entire volumes with discussions about raw food, vegetarianism, vitamins, etc. I should like to give the following advice to all people of the Occident who wish to practise Yoga for reasons of health but are not devoting themselves to it exclusively:

1. Let your food be natural and simple. In the beginning you can eat a mixed diet. The meatless diet of the Hindus is not a general rule, as *the necessity for eating meat is dependent upon climatic conditions*. In the tropics meat eating is dangerous, harmful, and entirely unnecessary. The colder the climate in which we live, the more justification there is for eating meat. For the population living in hot zones, the prohibition of eating meat has become a religious rule because it was desired to protect people who had no idea of hygiene from the injurious effects of a flesh diet. But what would happen to an Eskimo who for reasons of religious conviction decided to give up eating meat? He would simply starve: In the far north there are no coconuts, no bananas, and no pineapples, with their great nutritional value, to replace meat. The Eskimo is forced to eat blubber and drink seal fat in order to maintain his body temperature in the cruel arctic cold. For a person living in the tropics the mere thought of seal fat would be horrible. But were he transplanted to the arctic, he would quickly feel the same need and would soon lap up seal fat with the same relish as the Eskimo. Thus if an Eskimo decides to become a vegetarian—and in numerous vegetarian books I have read that only eaters of plants can expect to go to heaven! —he must simply emigrate to a warmer climate where fruit and green vegetables grow. I do not believe, however, that our heavenly Father reserves the salvation of the soul exclusively for the inhabitants of the warmer zones. The term 'mixed

diet' in Hatha Yoga means that meat should not be the basis but rather only an accompanying dish in the daily diet. Predominantly, we should eat fruit, vegetables, raw salads, milk, butter, and honey. One who can obtain these foods does best if he eats no meat at all. In the more advanced degrees of Yoga this is even a requirement. However, the Western pupil who is living in the world and starting in on the path of Yoga can eat meat, although seldom. He should eat more stone fruits and also give an honourable place in his regimen to onions and garlic. According to the ancient teachings of India and Tibet, garlic is the most excellent preventive for cancer. The occidental city dweller often lives his whole life without ever having eaten a single piece of this healthy vegetable, whereas a proper dietary is really unthinkable without it. For this reason, garlic may be ground fine and mixed with lemon juice in case anyone is afraid of being ostracized for eating it. I must also mention that rubbing the gums and the teeth with garlic or biting into onions and garlic in order to let their juices reach the roots of the teeth provides excellent protection against disorders such as gum bleeding and recession of the gums. In India the Brahmans teach their disciples: 'If you want to achieve wisdom, eat more onions.' Eating garlic also is recommended as a preventive for premature old age.

Finally I must mention a universal health food: the lemon. Everyone should eat at least one lemon daily, summer and winter. The most up-to-date rheumatism specialists prescribe the juice of two or three lemons daily, telling their patients to eat the grated rind mixed with honey. Unfortunately, lemons obtainable in northern countries are generally bitter, as they are picked before they are ripe. Their vitamin and medicinal value cannot compare with that of the exquisitely delicious, fully developed, tree-ripened fruit. It is therefore an advantage to mix the lemon juice with honey so as to prevent excessive acid from doing any harm.

2. The quantity of food must be in harmony with the requirements of the organism. It is unnecessary to repeat what I have already pointed out, namely, that we must adapt ourselves to the climatic and personal conditions. Everyone needs his individual special food; the person who

does physical work and the one who performs mental work. It makes a difference whether a person works outdoors or inside; there is a difference between a Yogi beginner and an initiate.

3. Meals should be eaten slowly, with attention, and concentration on the food. If we come home tired, we should rest at least ten minutes or a quarter of an hour; for a tired body has a tired stomach and cannot digest as it should. Moreover, let us not forget that food gives strength and that we should never eat when we are angry or dominated by another negative emotion. If we eat while in such a mental state, the energy derived from the food will serve to strengthen our anger and our baser instincts. On the contrary we should always eat with feelings of reverence, gratitude, and humility toward providence for supplying us with our food. In this way our mental and spiritual powers and our more noble characteristics will be enhanced. Saying grace at table is one of the religious rules found among all peoples of the world and it is a proof of the above mentioned truth.

Indians must take a bath and carefully wash hands and feet before their meals. They must also rinse out their mouths. For them this is a religious rule, but physicians know that it has a basis in hygiene, and they recommend it as a means of preserving the health. Modern occidental dietetic science agrees in almost all points with ancient Indian teachings. Advanced Yogi pupils are naturally bound by strict rules. They live near their master and are given instructions by him in these rules for healthy living. For Yoga pupils in the Occident, it is quite sufficient to follow those rules which call for moderation.

The occidental, according to my observation, makes the mistake of eating too much and too fast. Every mechanic knows that excessive heat and too much fuel prematurely wear out the machine and leave harmful residues behind. The impurities which collect in the body as a result of an improper diet, are eliminated from time to time through various diseases.

A typical cleansing disease is the one known in Europe as influenza (grippe). It would lead too far afield and exceed the scope of this book if I were to list in detail the precipitating causes of influenza. The fact is that nature uses high fever to burn out the wastes which have accumulated in the body and which do not belong there. At times also, these poisons are eliminated from the body through the formation of secretions or catarrh. This disease is here called influenza (grippe) and a predisposition towards it exists only amongst people who eat too much and eat predominantly of waste forming foods such as meat.

It is characteristic that in so-called 'good-times' when European populations were well nourished, influenza epidemics raged almost incessantly, whereas during the years of famine after the war, the disease disappeared almost entirely. During this time I was living in a country where the famine reached tremendous proportions and lasted a long time. To the best of human judgement, one could have assumed that a great epidemic would break out during the fall and winter among the debilitated inhabitants. On the contrary, influenza disappeared almost entirely. The people had not poisoned their blood by eating meat and too much food, so that the task of digesting and eliminating this excess from the body could not exceed the capacity of their organism. In spite of the fact that the entire population—with a few exceptions—spent the foggy, rainy, windy fall and winter with near-zero temperatures in unheated rooms and offices, there was no influenza. Thus too little nourishment seemed to be less injurious than too much!

The human organism can get along with surprisingly little food and can, when necessary, offset the nutritional deficiency through water and air. On the other hand, the body is unable to cope with an excess no matter how hard it may try to eliminate it. If we continue eating to excess, the uneliminated wastes are deposited within the body, and our organism is forced to clean house with catarrh and fever.

According to a Mohamedan Indian legend, Allah metes out to each person, when he is born, a certain amount of nourishment to last him through to the end of his days. If we consume this food too quickly, we die earlier. The more sparingly we eat, the longer we live.

In recommending moderation and a sober asceticism, the Mohamedan legend, the Christian Bible, the Lamas of Tibet, and the ancient teachings of the Indian Maharishis all agree.

91

— — — — —

IX

Kundalini and the Seven Chakras

IN the first chapter we mentioned the fact that our spine including the uppermost vertebra, the skull, is the carrier of life. In the uppermost curvature of the skull is the positive pole, while the lowest vertebra is the seat of the negative pole. The tension between both of them is what we call LIFE. The Yoga philosophy, many thousand years old, calls the positive pole the residence of the God Vishnu, the *spirit*; the negative pole, on the other hand, is the seat of Kundalini, the symbolically personified goddess of nature. Vishnu is the beaming fire and his brilliance constantly attracts Kundalini towards himself. Kundalini—coiled up like a snake in the lowest vertebra—waits for the moment when she can climb up through the channel of the spine and unite with her master Vishnu. The name Kundalini means the 'coiled one'.

This is the poetical and symbolical description of a physiological fact. In modern scientific language we would probably express it thus:

Between the positive pole in the skull and the negative pole in the lowest vertebra of the spine there is an electrical current of very short wave length. When the negative pole is freed from its normal location in the lowest vertebra and travels upward, it can reach the positive pole and unite with it. Whether we express ourselves symbolically or in scientific language, the fact remains that *this condition represents the highest fulfilment in consciousness and the most perfect realization of happiness. At that moment of union the eternal longing between the sexes is expressed in the highest fulfilment. The individual experiences within himself the supreme measure of perfection.*

This condition is known to the mystics all over the world. In the West it was called the 'mystic marriage' or the 'unio mystica'. Yoga exercises including pranayama, which tend to create perfect equilibrium, when practised in conjunction with certain asanas designed to awaken the negative pole, promote the 'union of Kundalini with Vishnu'. Kundalini and Vishnu each are located in an important nerve centre and between both of them there are several similar main nerve centres, each of which is a station for Kundalini to reach in her climb upward. When the energy which we call Kundalini advances upward and, one after the other, reaches each of these chakras, this always means a new step in consciousness on the way to finding one's SELF. These chakras are simply transformers and storage batteries for storing energy and prana. Most of these storage areas are dormant in the average person. The control of consciousness awakens these current centres—called chakras in Sanskrit—step by step in order that at the moment of fulfilment they are not overpowered, as this would injure the nervous system.

Fig. 5 facing page 94

Sometimes amongst people who have no understanding of Kundalini and the chakras and who are living on a very low plane of consciousness, some external impulse resulting from a blow or an accident may liberate Kundalini and cause it unexpectedly to race up the spinal column. As the consciousness of the average person is not dimensioned for this, he falls in a faint. In therapeutics this is called catalepsy. Whoever has consciously reached this condition with the aid of Yoga exercises will experience this supreme plane of consciousness ecstatically. For the spectator, he seems to be unconscious, as his consciousness has ascended to a higher plane. The individual himself, however, experiences this condition as a complete and perfect awakeness and awareness in consciousness, a state which is called 'blessedness' in the language of every religion. This is a physiological and psychic fact. It does not mean anything morbid but the complete, the perfect condition of man. There are seven main chakras and five smaller centres, making a grand total of twelve. In general, however, only the seven main chakras are named. The chakras are also called padmas (padma-lotus).

The seven main chakras are arranged in the following order one over the other.

The seat of Kundalini in the coccyx, in the lowest vertebra, is called

MULADHARA

This is a lotus with four leaves. The next one above it is

SVADHISHTHANA

in the nervous centre above the sexual organs. It is a lotus with six leaves. Then follows

MANIPURA

a ten-leaved lotus, in the nervous centre of the area of the navel.

ANAHATA

The chakra of the heart—a twelve-leaved lotus.

VISHUDDA

a chakra in the vicinity of the thyroid gland—the sixteen-leaved lotus.

AJNA

in the centre of the forehead between the two brows. It is a two-leaved lotus.

SAHASRARA

Vishnu—the seat of the positive pole at the top of the skull. A thousand-leaved lotus.

Along the spine there are three main channels called 'Nadi' in Sanskrit. On the left side is the negative 'Ida-Nadi'. On the right side, the positive 'Pingala-Nadi', and in the centre, in the marrow of the backbone, Sushumna-Nadi. This latter channel is the path of Kundalini.

In the lowest vertebra, Kundalini dwells in a triangular chakra. Through concentrated exercises the Yogi brings her from one chakra to the next, higher and higher, until she reaches Sahasrara. Each new chakra reached opens up a new condition of consciousness for the Yogi. He comes into the possession of clear vision, the art of reading thoughts, of having visions of a high order, or surveying the past, present and future, and of further occult faculties, depending on the chakra which is activated, until he reaches the condition of complete illumin-

94

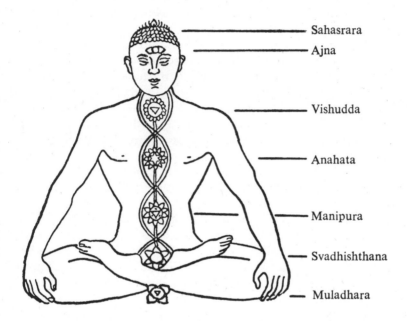

Sahasrara

Ajna

Vishudda

Anahata

Manipura

Svadhishthana

Muladhara

FIG. 5

ation, the union of Kundalini with Vishnu. This is the highest plane, the level on which the individual consciousness fuses and becomes one with the OVERSELF, with God. The basis of every religion is the secret which lies hidden within the spine of each individual, and which does not rest on imagination, but is actually the most *perfect truth itself*.

This fulfilment is called samadhi by the Yogis. Although this pertains to Raja Yoga, the final goal of spiritual Yoga, it was necessary to mention it here as the condition of illumination is not only a spiritual but also physiological fact. The awakening of the chakras from their latent condition to consciousness is also the purpose of Hatha Yoga exercises. If the chakra exercises are practised incorrectly they can become very dangerous; their practice without a responsible teacher is therefore not permissible. However, we shall not discuss this further, as this is a matter for the advanced Yogi pupil who is called a 'chela'. The various paths followed by Yoga cannot be separated by a sharp dividing line any more than the body from the mind. The body is the structure, the clothing, the frame, and carrier of the mind. Our complete knowledge of the body leads us to the mind and the latter to the OVERSELF.

From the foregoing it is obvious that the effect of Hatha Yoga exercises is so many-sided and so all inclusive that it is worth while for everyone who is trying to progress to devote his careful attention to Hatha Yoga whether he does so for reasons of health or in order to reach higher spiritual results—for we must always remember the ancient admonition: a healthy mind in a healthy body.

ILLUSTRATIONS

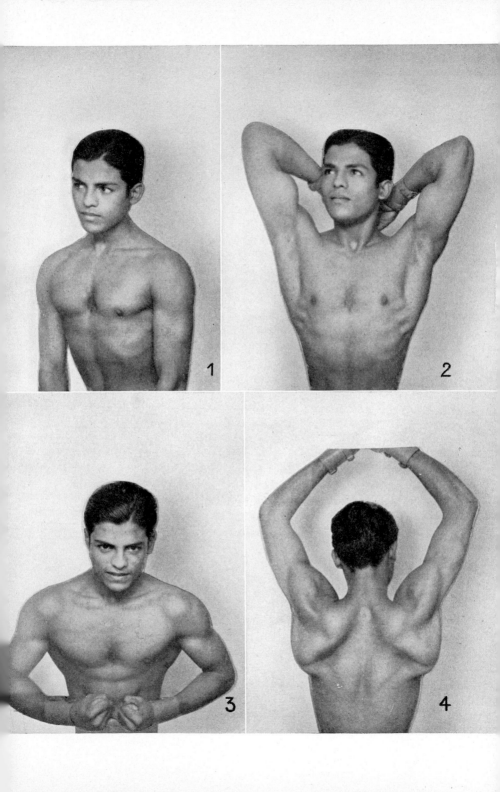

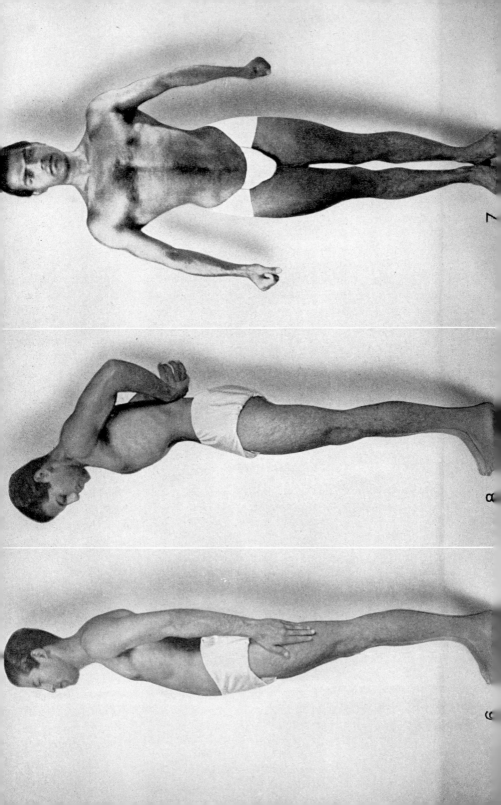

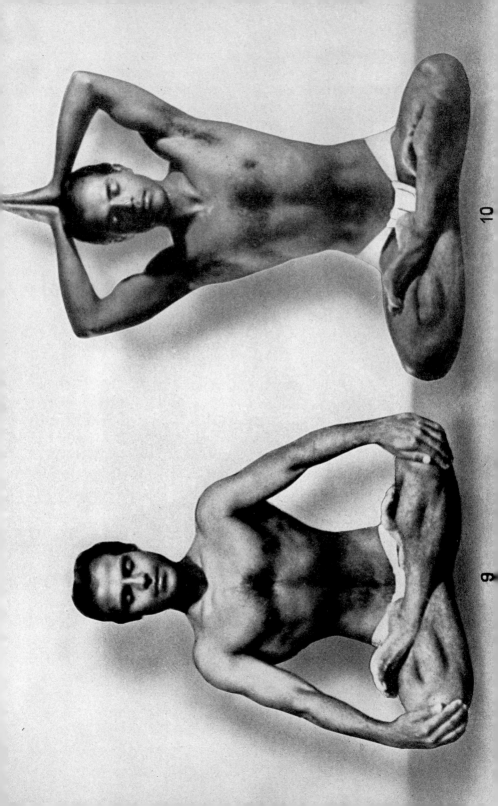

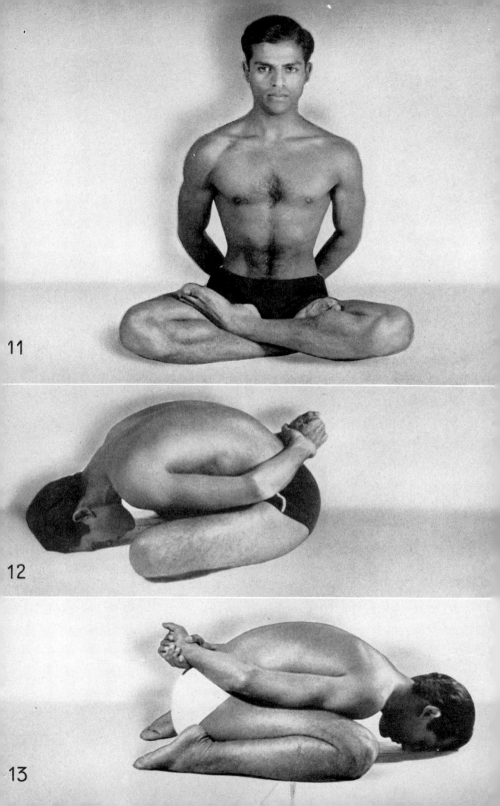

11

12

13

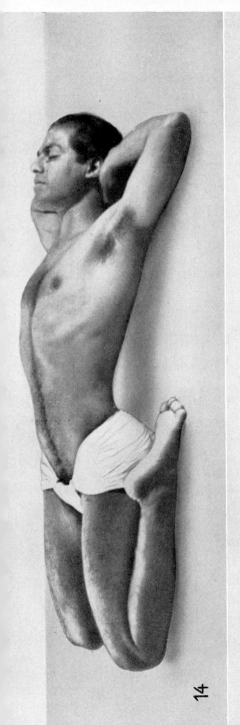

14

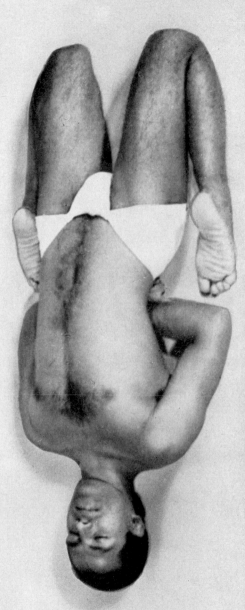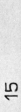

15

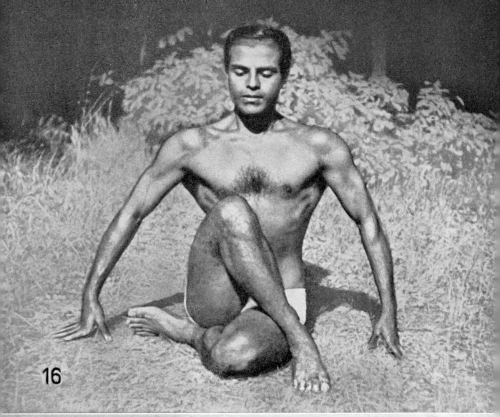

16

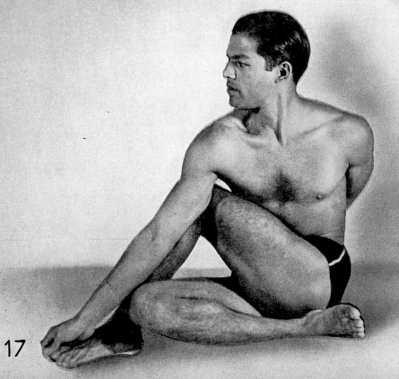

17

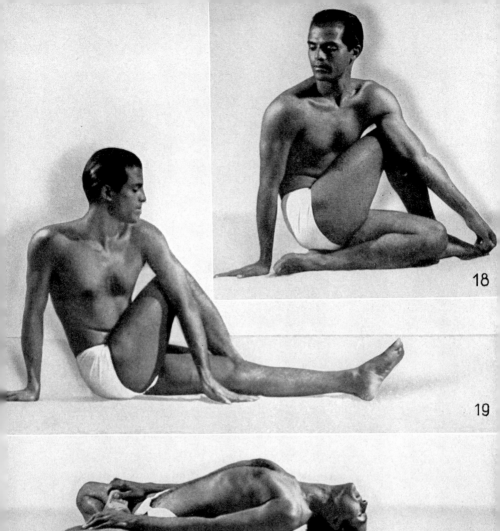

18

19

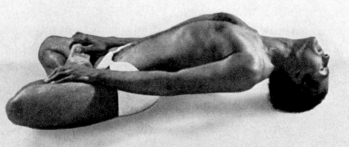

20

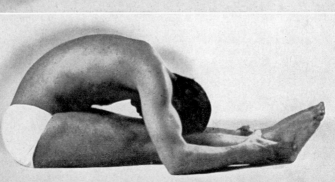

21

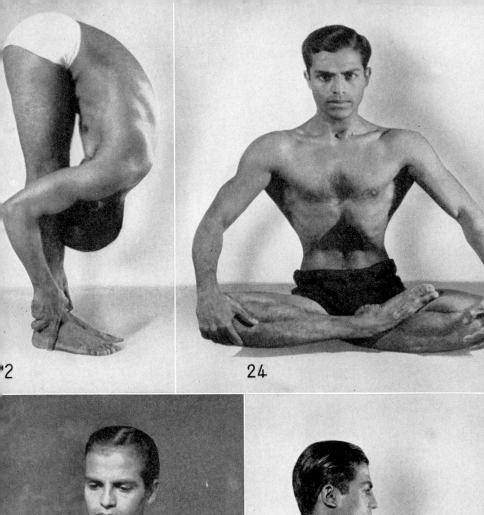

2

24

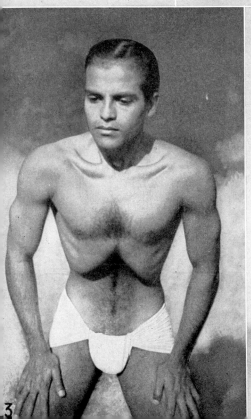

3

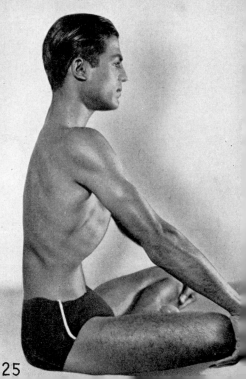

25

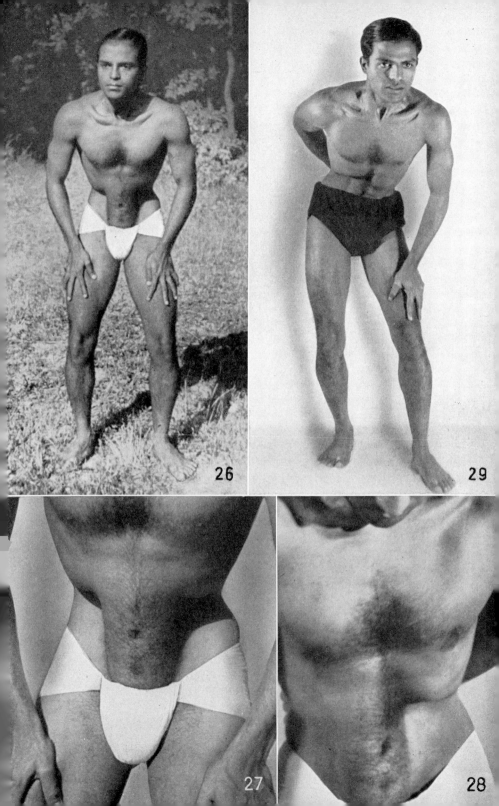

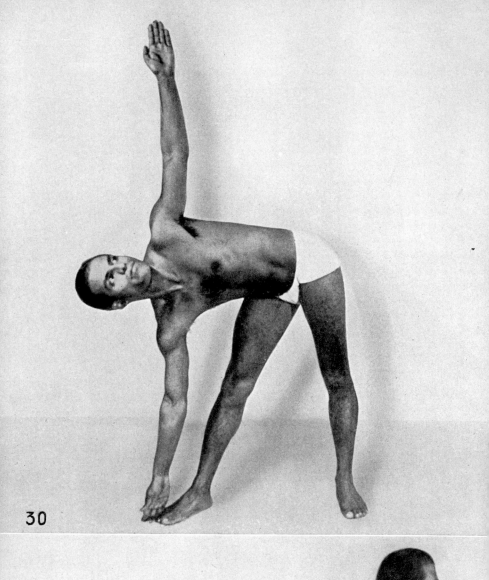

30

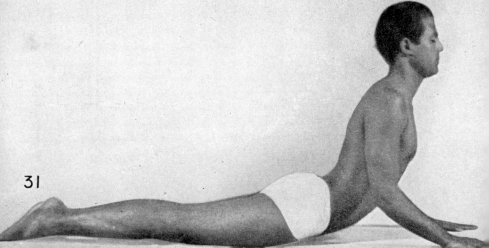

31

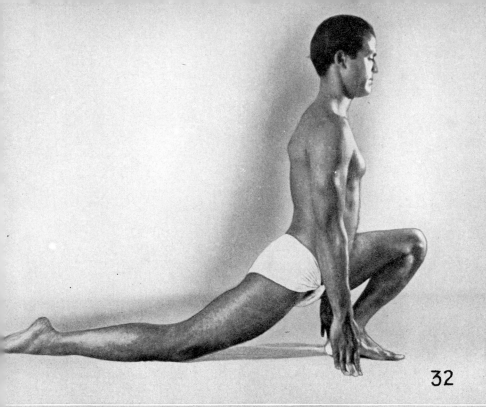

32

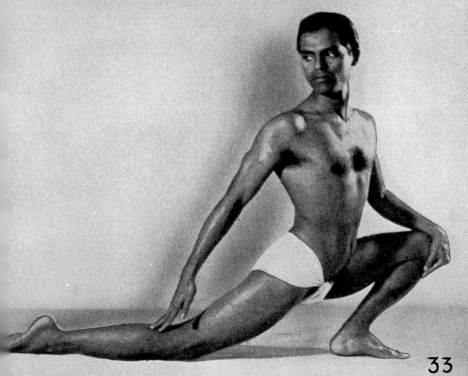

33

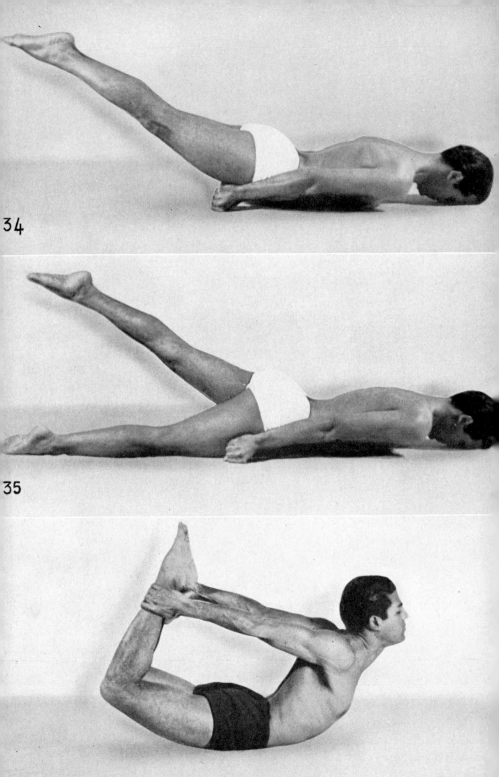

34

35

36

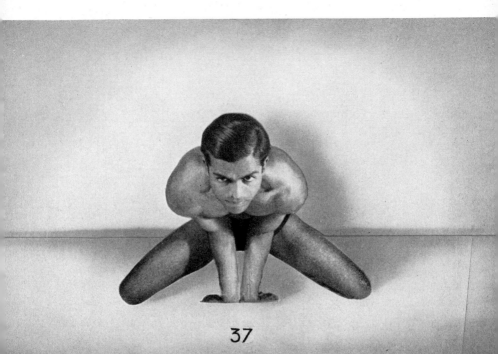

37

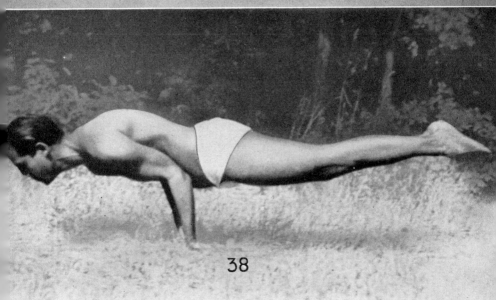

38

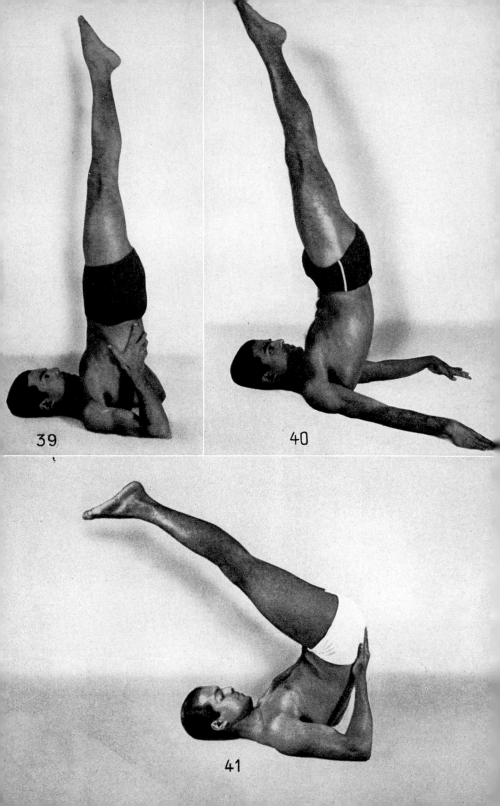

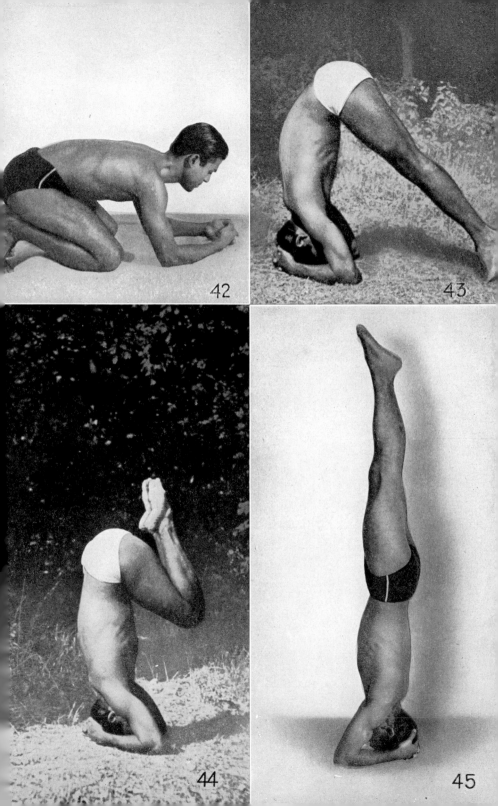

42

43

44

45

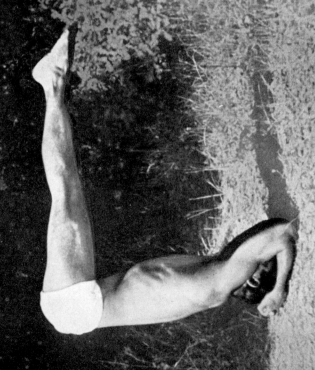

46

48

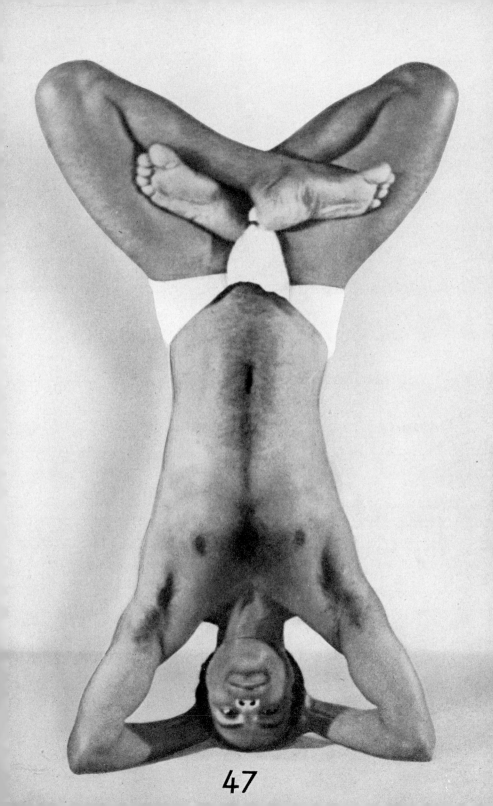

47

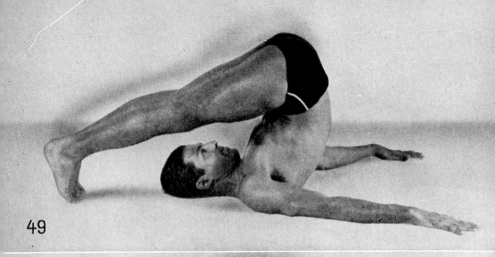

49

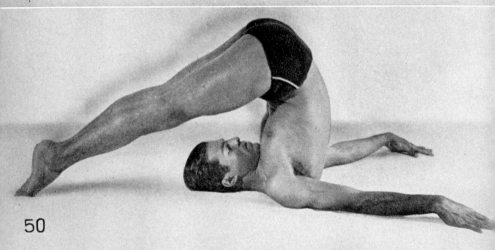

50

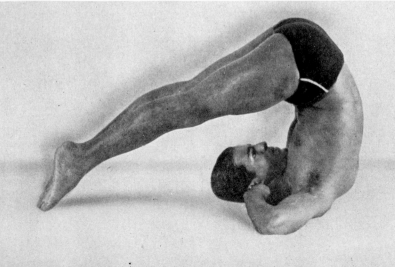

51

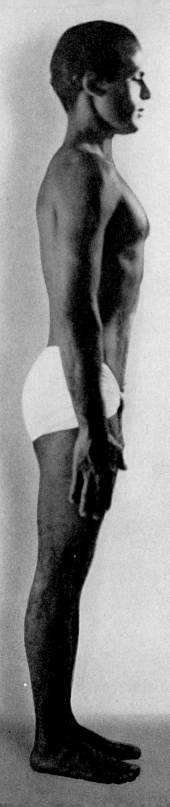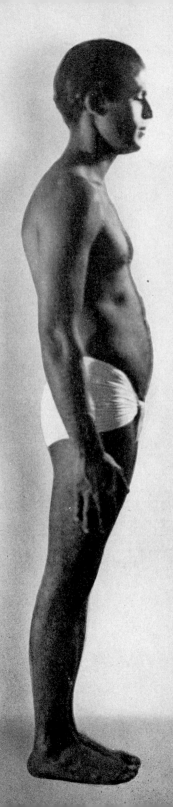

52

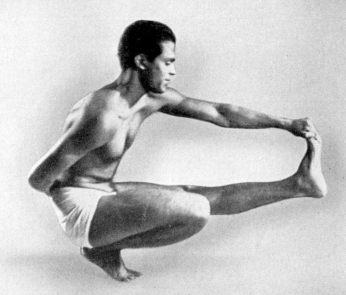

53

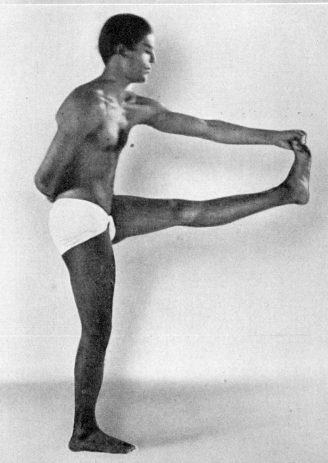

54

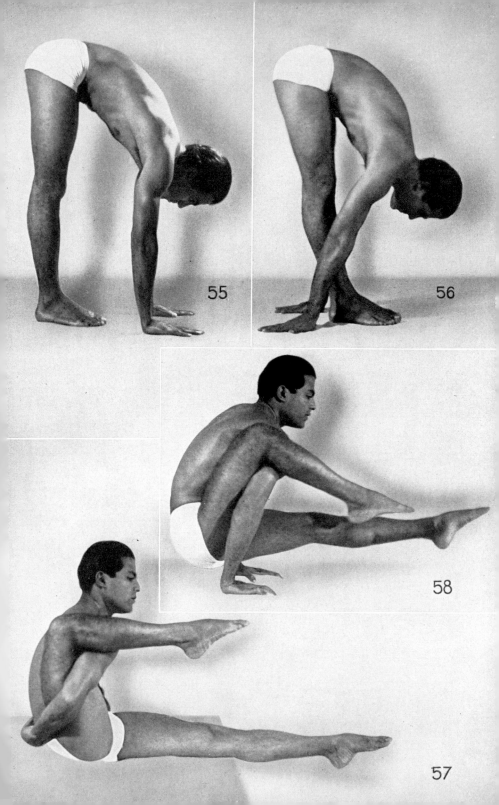

55

56

58

57

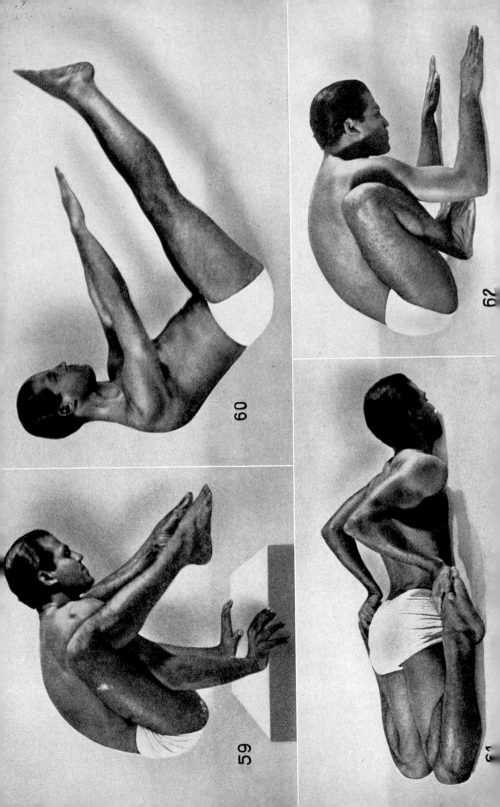

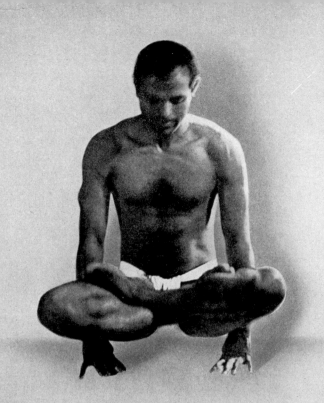

63

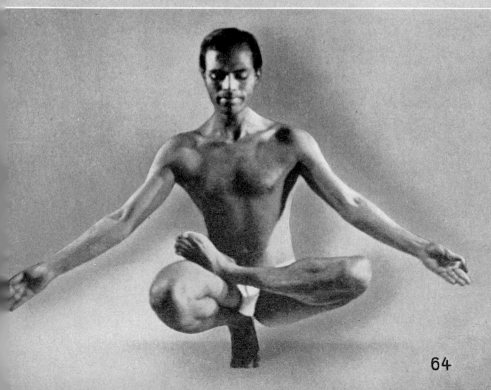

64

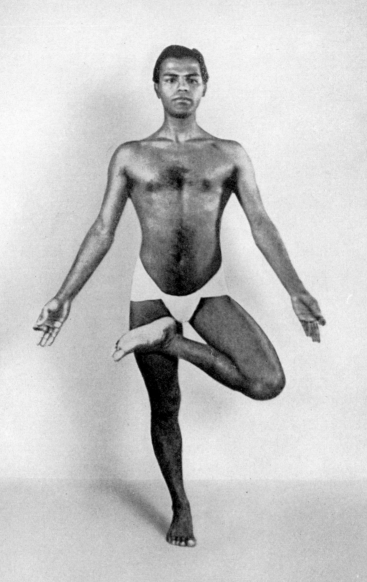

65

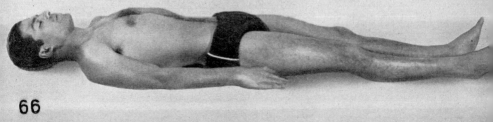

66

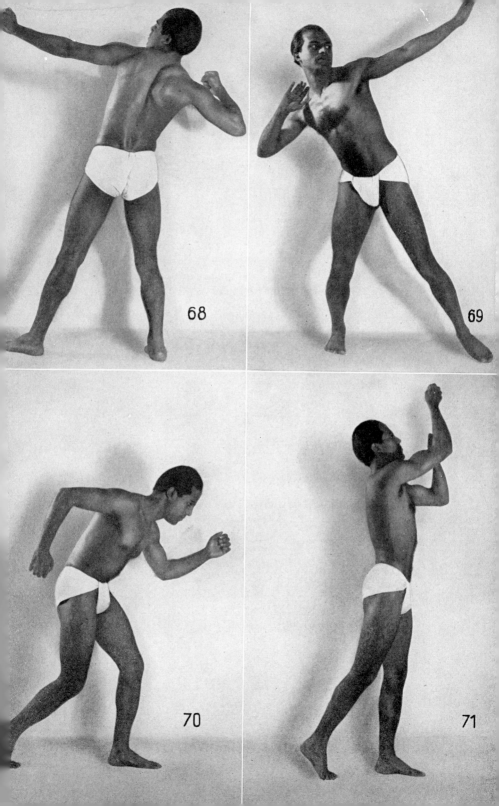

68

69

70

71

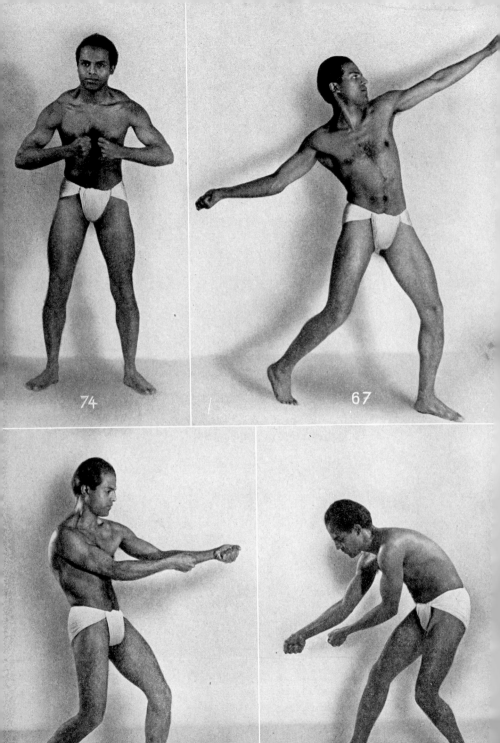

74

67

73

72

PART 2

_ _ _ _ _ _ _ _

Practical Hatha Yoga

X

————

The Constructive Power
of Consciousness

EXERCISES of Hatha Yoga consist of three parts: the control of consciousness, breath control (pranayama), and physical postures (asanas).

The three must be exercised jointly for one is not thinkable without the other two. The control of consciousness cannot be exercised without a certain body posture and without breathing, and I can likewise not breathe or hold my body in any position without consciousness, at least in my head if not elsewhere. The Hatha Yoga exercises prescribe exactly how the three are to be combined if I wish my development to be steady and lead to greater and greater results.

For this reason the exercises are grouped and each is named according to the point which is primarily emphasized among the three practical factors. Our main goal is to direct the consciousness to all parts of the body equally, or in other words to animate our body completely. This gives us the key to the control over the positive and negative energies. In exercising we get acquainted with the power of consciousness. We even attain the ability to produce currents of energy at will and direct them to any point of our body through simple concentration of thought.

The permanent seat of our consciousness is the grey matter. It would be wearisome and go beyond the scope of this book to discuss how the innermost cells of the grey matter differ from all other nerve cells. This belongs in technical books on medicine. *The essential fact of importance for us is that, through the constant influence of the* SELF, *the cells of the grey matter have developed into the perfect instrument they now are.* The SELF entered the brain cells, took possession of them, and developed them into obedient tools. If, by an act of our will, we send our consciousness to other nerve cells, the latter begin to develop and can also become just as perfect carriers of consciousness as the highest cells of the grey matter. What is to prevent me, therefore, from leading my SELF into any part of my body at will, when this part contains nerve cells with the same properties as those of the grey matter? Countless examples prove that the duties of an important nerve, if the latter is destroyed by an accident, are taken over by another nerve. The adaptability and elasticity of the nerves is confirmed in a way that often borders on the miraculous; the Hatha Yogi merely makes use of these abilities.

Through long practice, consciousness can develop every nerve cell to a higher ability and make it the conductor of a current of a higher order. Naturally time is necessary to accomplish this. One who has the gift of concentration can himself achieve the above-mentioned result. As soon as he directs his consciousness to the nerve cells of one part of his body a *reaction is immediately caused.* Naturally this reaction is not so great that the bundle of nerves concerned could be used right away for *thinking.* At present we must be satisfied when, as a result of the higher currents directed to them, these nerves are stimulated and we feel a prickly sensation of warmth and a circulation of blood. If, however, we direct our consciousness daily—unceasingly for years—to a group of nerves, the latter begin to develop and step by step become able to transmit the higher manifestations of the SELF. Thus, little by little, we can animate every part of our body and make it conscious. . . .

Advanced Yogis are able at will to accelerate or bring to a standstill their digestive processes or the activity of their heart. In the literature of the world we can find numerous examples of fakirs who have permitted themselves to be buried for weeks at a time. And a famous case was that of a Yogi who for purely scientific purposes submitted to a dangerous experiment under the strictest control at the medical faculty in Madras. He swallowed a large dose of cyanide and conducted the poison intact through his digestive tract, without the slightest bit

100

being absorbed by his body. The poison then left his body in the natural way.

Awakening the consciousness, in addition to its tremendous importance for the health, has another great advantage. It helps to *assure us that consciousness also exists independently of the brain. Consciousness is not the product of the brain*—as the materialist would have us believe—*but the reasoning of the* SELF, *the 'I', which exists independently of matter. Yoga exercises lead us to the experience of immortality, because we become acquainted with the Master of the body, the eternal* SELF, *which stands beyond perishableness.*

A large part of humanity is plagued by conscious or unconscious fear of death. How many healthy people are chronically paralysed by the thought ever lying in wait in the back of their mind, 'What's the use of all of this if in the end there is unavoidably cnly destruction . . . death?'—Yoga completely heals us from this fear.

To those who insist upon tangible proof I recommend their taking the trouble and making the experiment. If for example someone cannot stand on his head, he can see for himself that others who are stronger and have better mastery of equilibrium can perform this trick. Mental experiences, however, occur in the depth of the mind and are invisible for others. The SELF is invisible and there is no instrument in the world with the aid of which its existence could be proved. *Only in its effect can we feel the* SELF *of another person. We will get acquainted with our own* SELF *when we develop the consciousness and become conscious of our* SELF. The immortal higher SELF—invisible for everyone else—can only be experienced on the inside. The Yogi sits immovably while he experiences conditions of consciousness of a higher order; if we want to get acquainted with the results which he achieves through concentration, we must also *experience the same thing.* The Yogi can only do one thing in order to prove his truth: *he shows us the way.*

For anyone who does not believe in the miraculous effect of consciousness upon the body I recommend the following simple experiment. Let him hold his right hand, fist clenched, with his index finger extended. Now let him direct his consciousness to the index finger; that is, let him think with his entire concen-

101

tration focused on the extended finger, with the feeling that he *is going into the point of the finger*. After a short time he will feel a strong prickling and warmth. Little by little the finger will be pulsed through by warmth and if his concentration is strong enough, the warmth will increase to a boiling heat. However, not only warmth but blood circulation is the result and little by little the finger will get red. If through steady practice we achieve mastery of the control of consciousness, we can immediately derive great benefit from it. We can prevent a cold, for example, if in rainy, windy, weather we concentrate intently on our feet. Positive energy and warmth can be created in this way and we can thus prevent our feet from getting so cold that bacilli get the upper hand. Similarly, if our back is cold, and if our back muscles are already conscious, we can, by concentrating our muscles produce more energy and thus avoid pneumonia.

With keen pleasure I have observed that my European pupils are very receptive to the matter of control of consciousness. In countless cases, by this very simple method, they have achieved complete healing even in serious cases of freezing, disturbances of the circulation, digestive disorders, and even in apparently incurable cases of paralysis. The nerve which has almost been destroyed by long lasting inflammation is no longer able to carry the current of life and the part of the body concerned is lifeless or paralysed. Consciousness, however, is the strongest awakening and animating power. It is even more valuable than electricity and massage. If our concentration is strong enough, the consciousness breaks through the insulation, the nerve recovers its efficiency, and healing results.

One who understands the meaning of leading consciousness also understands the advantages that are connected with being able to cause a flow of blood to any desired part of his body. If someone suffers from a lazy colon, he concentrates on his colon and feels *as if he himself were the colon*. This in itself is sufficient to cause a flow of blood and to set the colonic activity in motion. This is increased when the person imagines *that he himself is the colon and moving*. Anyone who has tried this even a single time could feel that his body obeyed immediately and adapted itself to the imagination. Those who have not succeeded in controlling their consciousness at the first attempt, *should not despair.* Repeated attempts will bring fruit, and this in turn will strengthen their will power. *There is no greater joy than the victory of the* SELF *over matter, over the body.*

Parallel with the guiding of consciousness, pranayama exercises and the various body postures (called asanas in Sanskrit) are a great help in the awakening of the body.

The importance of breath control from the physiological point of view has already been discussed in the first part of this book. In the guiding of consciousness this regulation of breath is also very important. During inhalation we must concentrate on storing up prana within ourselves, and in exhaling we must think of sending forth the fresh prana intentionally to all parts of the body or to the part which is concerned in the particular exercise. Thus in the exercise called *Viparita-Karani* we concentrate on the thyroid gland. This means, that we send our SELF into the thyroid gland,—through constantly thinking of it—and simultaneously at every exhalation we send the quantity of prana we have inhaled to the thyroid, much as if we were 'pumping it there'.

Similarly we can send prana to any desired part of the body with the firm intention of strengthening or healing it. Prana collects wherever the consciousness is concentrated. Where the light shines, the moths collect!

Naturally, our body becomes the strongest and will work most intensively in the place where we concentrate our consciousness, as this induces the greatest flow of prana to the part concerned. The scientist holds his consciousness in his brain, and the greatest amount of prana collects there, hence his brain will develop and increase in efficiency. The wrestler or boxer constantly concentrates his attention, that is his consciousness, on the grip of his hands and the blows of his fists. The muscles grow due to the prana collecting there.

Among animals the same condition applies, corresponding to the animal's degree of consciousness. The hare is always afraid of the attacks of stronger animals. It therefore listens intently and pricks up its ears at every sound. As a result, the attention fixed in its ears has caused the greatest amount of prana to collect there, and inasmuch as prana is the constructive force, its ears and organs of hearing, in the course of millions of years, have

103

grown relatively very long and become an infinitely fine instrument.

Under similar rules everything alive develops, including plants, animals, and man. Prana works constructively wherever it is sent by the consciousness. Thus there came into being the trunk of the elephant, the neck of the giraffe, the legs of the ostrich, the innumerable variations in the animal kingdom, and thus also *man has developed into the creature he now is*. Man, however, has not yet reached perfection. He still carries an infinity of possibilities within himself. Prana thus *automatically* follows the consciousness. How much more we could achieve if we would exploit this natural law and *knowingly* and systematically exercise the control of prana. If we do not know the secrets and laws of our being, we are in constant danger of committing errors through ignorance, thus making our body sick. We must therefore learn the laws of guiding prana and radiating our consciousness into the body. Then we have obtained the key to perfect health and long life.

One who makes a conscious act out of his breathing and follows the path of the air in the lungs will, step by step, become more receptive and capable of perception. Little by little he will be able to feel the fine current of prana. Afterwards he will get acquainted with the main bundle of nerves which conduct prana into the storage and distributing centres, the chakras. It is no longer a secret for us that the chakras are located in the main nerve centres and the most important ductless glands. If the wrong current or an inadequate one reaches them, sooner or later they will suffer. And because the normal functioning of the other organs depends on these centres, any such disturbances can bring on the most diverse disorders. Thus it is of the greatest importance to preserve—or reacquire—the health of these main centres. Here, in addition to guiding of consciousness and regulation of breath, Hatha Yoga physical exercises play a very important part.

— — — — —

XI

Therapeutic Effect of the Ancient Asanas

THE origin of the Yoga postures known as 'asanas' is lost in the mists of ancient Indian legend. According to these sources, the god Shiva demonstrated 84,000 postures in order to show the physical exercises which were suitable for maintaining human health and attaining a higher degree of self knowledge. Of these postures, eighty-four are in common use today, and the number used to preserve or recover health amounts to from twenty to thirty. Even if they did not originate with the god Shiva, these asanas were developed by *rishis* and *maharishis*, the great wise men of India, the Yogis of a higher order who were masters of the most marvellous physiological, physical and so-called 'super-natural' sciences. The postures have come down through the centuries in the form in which they are now crystallized. Seventy or even fifty years ago Occidental scientists would have shrugged off this series of asanas as a superstition. Today, however, in my own experience, the most incredulous European who is interested in his physical wellbeing recognizes the extraordinary importance of these postures, particularly since the most up-to-date western medical scientists have demonstrated their effect through experiments.

Aside from postures which are primarily used for meditation, pranayama, and mudras (exercises for persistence and concentration), the so-called physical postures (asanas) are of the utmost benefit for the organism. There is no praise that is too great when we come to describe *the almost supernatural effect of the physical postures on the human organism and their role in*

105

the preservation of vital force and the promotion of health. It was not until recently that the Indian Yoga research institutes, with the co-operation of reputable European therapeutic scientists, were able to discover the medical secrets behind the Indian asanas.

It is a well-known physiological fact that the health of the human body depends on the condition of the cells and tissues. In order to be healthy, the tissues need:

1. *Regular food intake and perfect functioning of the internal secretion glands (endocrines);*
2. *Rapid and thorough elimination of wastes from the organism;*
3. *Healthy and perfect functioning of the nervous system.*

Thus it is clear that the digestive and circulatory system must be in perfect condition in order to be able to provide the tissues with protein, sugar, fat, salts, and other important materials. Let us now investigate how the asanas affect the organs of digestion and the circulation of the blood.

Let us first examine the *effect of the asanas on the digestive system.* The digestive organs—stomach, small intestines, the pancreas gland, liver, etc., are contained in the abdominal cavity which is supported beneath by the pelvis and on the sides by strong muscles. Mother nature has provided for these organs to receive a gentle and regular massage through the rise and fall of the diaphragm in breathing. This promotes their functioning. Every minute the organs of digestion receive about forty to fifty automatic massages which are indispensable to the maintenance of health.

As we have shown in the chapter on the regulation of breath, civilized city-dwelling human beings cannot breathe properly. This means that their breathing has so degenerated and their abdominal muscles are so stunted that the insufficient massaging of the organs of digestion causes a disturbance in the secretion of stomach acid. Digestive disturbances and, very frequently, serious stomach troubles are the result. The exercise of pranayama is not sufficient in itself for people with defective breathing and degenerated abdominal muscles. Such persons must resort to asanas in order to recover the complete health of their abdominal organs. The asanas not only supply these organs

106

with an external massage, but also give them a unique internal exercise which cannot be equalled by any other system of sports in the world. It is a recognized fact of therapeutics that the muscles can only retain their strength and elasticity if they are obliged to perform contracting and stretching movements. Among the asanas *Bhujangasana, Salabhasana,* and *Dhanurasana* are some of the most magnificent exercises for stretching the abdominal muscles and contracting the back muscles. *Yoga Mudra, Paschimotasana, Padahastasana* and *Halasana,* on the other hand, contract the abdominal muscles and stretch the muscles of the back. *Vakrasana* and *Ardha-Matsyendrasana* exercise the lateral muscles of the abdomen. *Salabhasana* is the most perfect exercise for the lungs and the muscles of the back.

The beauty of Yoga exercises, however, is most apparent in the asanas *Uddiyana* and *Nauli.* Although these two are among the most difficult asanas, their mastery is worth all the effort necessary as they are of most astounding effect on the abdominal muscles as well as on the internal organs. The first mentioned exercise massages the external and internal muscles vertically while the second performs this work laterally. But the strength of the abdominal muscles is not only important for the regular massaging of the internal organs, but also in order to keep these organs in their proper places in the abdominal cavity. These organs hang freely in the abdominal cavity or are attached loosely to its back wall; hence the need for a strong support in front to prevent the abdominal organs from slipping out of place (prolapse of the stomach, intestines, kidneys, vagina, etc.). Thus the Yoga postures not only maintain the elasticity of the abdominal muscles and the organs in the abdominal cavity through their automatic massage, but they also help support them in their proper place.

As the circulation of the blood serves to carry food particles from the organs of digestion to the tissues, *a healthy circulatory system is of capital importance.* The most important organ of circulation is the heart which, as we well know, has the strongest muscle. Even the muscles of the heart can be made more resistant and stronger through Yoga exercises. Uddiyana and Nauli massage the heart from below through the raising of the diaphragm. We must also remember that a muscle can be kept

107

in perfect condition by subjecting it to alternating pressures. The heart, however, lies in the mediastinum and every increase or decrease in pressure necessarily affects it. Bhujangasana, Salabhasana, Dhanurasana, Sarvangasana, Viparita-Karani, and Halasana all subject the heart to alternating pressure during the first part of the exercise and thus actively promote the health of the organs of circulation.

Of all the organs of circulation, the veins are the weakest. Nevertheless, they are obliged to collect the blood in all the various parts of the body and, against the pull of gravity, to conduct it back to the heart. This 'up-hill' work puts the greatest burden on the weak walls of the veins; hence the complaints we hear about 'varicose veins'. The veins need external help even more than the other organs of circulation. Even thousands of years ago the wise men and teachers in India knew that the blood vessels can be strengthened by exercises such as Sirshasana, Sarvangasana, and Viparita-Karani which, because of the inverted position of the body, enable the blood to flow back to the heart without effort. These postures which reduce the pressure on the veins for several minutes every day tend to lengthen the life of the veins to a considerable degree. Their effect is astonishing. The short rest which these blood vessels obtain during the exercise of the asanas is fully adequate for their regeneration. With daily asana exercises of several minutes' duration, even varicose veins can be cured. This is not so un-believable as it may sound when we consider the tremendous ability of the human organism to regenerate itself when it is given healthy conditions. Moreover, we must not neglect the proper nutrition of the tissues and the intake of oxygen. In the chapters about breathing we have already discussed the in-creasing of the oxygen turnover in the body and the vitalizing and life-prolonging effect of lung exercises. In this connection we should merely like to mention that through the practice of Yoga asanas, the muscles of the thorax are even further strengthened, and the results of pranayama combined with asanas are even more apparent. Salabhasana is the quintessence of perfect lung exercise, and for this reason it is also called 'pranayama-asana'. In exercising Salabhasana the air must be sucked in deeply and held under high lung pressure for a few seconds until the end of the exercise. Through practising **Salab-hasana** two or three times every day, even the smallest lung alveolus and every last cell of the lungs will be improved and strengthened by the mighty rhythm of breathing.

The asanas have a cleansing effect on the air passages, so that certain body postures supplement pranayama. In very many cases they protect us from tonsilitis and colds. *Sarvangasana, Viparita-Karani, Matsyasana, Jivabandha* and *Simhamudra* are magnificent preventives to curb incipient tonsilitis, and they can even cure colds.

The health of the tissues and hence the health of the entire human organism not only depends on proper and systematic food supply, but also—as we have mentioned at the beginning of this chapter—on the perfect functioning of the *internal secretion (endocrine) glands.* The pineal, thyroid, pituitary, suprarenal, sexual glands, etc., are the most important endocrine glands in the organism. The inadequate or deficient functioning of any one of these glands can cause the most serious disorders. The following asanas are excellently suited for maintaining the health of the thyroid: *Sarvangasana, Viparita-Karani, Matsyasana, Jivabandha and Simhamudra.* The pituitary and pineal glands are benefited by *Sarvangasana,* and the sexual glands by *Sarvangasana, Uddiyana and Nauli.*

The second prerequisite for the health of the tissues is the complete elimination of wastes: carbon dioxide, uric acid, urine, faeces, and perspiration. If for any reason these toxic substances remain in the body longer than necessary, they can cause serious disorders. They can only be efficiently eliminated when the organs of breathing, elimination of water and digestion function perfectly.

I have already mentioned the asanas which beneficially effect breathing and digestion. The health of the kidneys is promoted by *Uddiyana, Nauli, Bhujanagasana* and *Dhanurasana.*

The third prerequisite for the health of the tissues is the perfect functioning of the nervous system.

The most important part of the nervous system is the brain, followed by the mighty nerve cord in the spinal column and the two lines of nerves in the sympathetic system. From the brain and the spinal column, the nerves branch out to all parts of the body. This network of nerves is so complete that there is not a single part of tissue anywhere in the body which is not in contact with the nervous system. If for any reason the nerves deteriorate, the tissues will function inadequately, and if the nerve connections to a given part of the body cease to work or if they are destroyed, that part is paralysed. If the nerves of the large intestine degenerate, the large intestine will cease functioning properly and the result is constipation or chronic intestinal catarrh. If we cut one of the nerves of the face or if it is paralysed, the muscles served by this nerve can no longer contract.

The ancient system of Indian postures has just as beneficial an effect on the nervous system as on the organs of digestion, the endocrine glands, and the organs of elimination. *Sirshasana* and *Viparita-Karani* also serve to carry a richer supply of blood to the brain and thus provide more oxygen to nerves serving the organs of sense. In this connection the Yoga exercises place the greatest emphasis on the muscles of the abdomen and the backbone. In strengthening the latter and the muscles which serve it, we simultaneously build up the nerves running through the spinal column, together with the bundles of sympathetic nerves. Similarly the other asanas strengthen the nerves of the thorax, the abdomen, the back, and the sides. Through supplying fresh blood to the head, the appropriate asanas promote the mental faculties (memory, ambition, enjoyment of work, etc.) and help us to achieve self-control. Those who wish to exercise mental Yoga, i.e., Raja Yoga, will do well, therefore, to begin their exercises with Hatha Yoga.

It should be pointed out that, though the asanas are capable of maintaining the body and muscles in health and strength, they are not suitable for developing mighty muscles and an athletic looking body. Persons who not only wish to achieve perfect health, but also desire to build large and powerful muscles can easily achieve this goal through another branch of Yoga combined with slow motion exercises. From the European point of view, this is a completely new and novel system of muscular exercise. It is described in a later chapter.

The complete description of the asanas and the introduction to their practical exercise is also contained in one of the following chapters. Let us not forget, however, that the exercise of the asanas always requires a peaceful mental state. If we begin our work in a happy mood and a settled frame of mind, the healing forces set free by the exercises need not be used up to neutralize negative emotional feelings but can immediately begin their marvellous calming effect on our nerves. The meditative posture which is assumed before the beginning of the asanas serves this purpose. The pupil should always endeavour to forget his problems and all the difficulties of life simply by turning his thoughts towards the higher moral code of Yama and Niyama.

'Believe in the creator and you will believe in your own strength. Be just, and life will be just to you!—Be moderate in all expressions of your life and then you will live long on earth!— Be calm with the calmness of the morning. Believe in the future as you believe in the sunrise. Regard the world with a happy tranquillity! For after all, He who made and preserves the world has a watchful eye on you too!' With such thoughts we create a clear atmosphere in and about us and can then begin our exercises.

_ _ _ _ _

XII

Pranayama and Asanas
THE SECRET OF LONG LIFE

ON the basis of the practical description of Yoga asanas and a comparison of these prescriptions with the chapters on pranayama, it will not appear incredible to any open minded pupil of the Occident that through regulation of breath and with the aid of the ancient Yoga exercises, everyone can prolong his life.

Moreover, we shall present here an exact description of the most important breathing exercises and asanas, explain how each one is executed, and instruct the reader regarding the mental and physical benefits derived therefrom. Like all physical exercises, Hatha Yoga is only beneficial when it is applied intelligently. Just as boxing, running, swimming, tennis and other sports can be harmful if they are indulged in to excess or if we disregard the rules of health (exercising with a full stomach on a very hot day, for example), in a like manner the improper practice of Hatha Yoga can be very dangerous, particularly because Hatha Yoga exercises are powerfully effective. Properly practised, however, their effect is beneficial! On the other hand if we perform Hatha Yoga exercises injudiciously and allow ourselves to be carried away to excesses through not taking proper account of our present circumstances, the harm can be just as great. Experience shows, however, that one who observes even to a slight extent the reaction of his own organism, soon feels instinctively which exercises are beneficial to him and which ones might harm him; then he will select the ones that benefit him most. No one who is suffering from disorders of the lungs, kidneys, heart, liver or similar conditions should exercise without the instruction of a competent teacher! The healthy pupil will doubtless be able to judge which exercises are of benefit to him and which should better be avoided. In case of congestion or when he has a full stomach, he will not exercise Viparita-Karani or Sirshasana; neither will he exercise Uddiyana-Bandha or Nauli when he has an acutely upset stomach or intestinal catarrh.—On the other hand, in cases of cerebral anaemia, haemorrhoids or varicose veins, he will have recourse to Sarvangasana. Etc.

By way of illustration, a table based on long years of experience is given at the end of this book. A pupil who follows this table closely is bound to benefit from his exercises. We warn our readers most emphatically, however, not to be misled by the apparent simplicity of the initial exercises. No one should feel that any of them are 'too easy' and can be skipped. Such a procedure would be very unwise. Exercises involving retention of the breath, when such retention is begun gently and gradually prolonged, are beneficial, but excesses in this regard can lead to dilation of the lungs or heart.

One Yogi pupil in India, for example, was told by his master— by way of introduction—to do seven full Yogi breathings in the morning, at noon, and in the evening. 'Seven exercises are not enough for me,' thought the pupil. 'Seven probably won't even have any effect at all!' In order to progress more quickly he did the exercise *fifty times*. By the next day, his body had broken out all over with a red rash. The teacher explained to him that his strained breathing had resulted in a rapid stirring up of all the impurities and toxins in his body and this toxic matter had been driven into his skin in the form of a rash. For a day or two he suffered from a high temperature and an excruciating itch until his condition returned to normal. From then on the over-ambitious pupil was content to progress at the rate prescribed by his teacher! So let us take our time and exercise with patience in accordance with wise instructions based on thousands of years of experience. Then there can be no disturbances and we will feel *only the beneficial effect of Hatha Yoga*.

In the tables the exercises are so arranged that an invigorating exercise is always followed by a relaxing, strengthening, or restful one. For the uninitiated beginner in the Occident it is thus worth while to follow the table exactly.

113

It is best to perform the exercises early in the morning or in the evening before supper,—never with a full stomach! Likewise, it is not recommended to exercise immediately before going to bed, as the quantities of oxygen and prana absorbed during pranayama and the stimulating asanas have such a freshening effect that it is difficult to go to sleep after performing them.

XIII

_ _ _ _ _

Pranayama Breathing Exercises

THE most important prerequisite for regulation of breathing is
to control the rhythm. For this reason we must always remember
to breathe regularly, counting out exactly the prescribed rhythm.
To measure the time, Indian Yogis count their pulse beats.
The best procedure is to take our pulse and determine the rhythm
of the heart beat before beginning the exercises. This rhythm is
the basis of our counting. Every breathing exercise is begun with a
vigorous exhalation.

The basis of breathing exercises is the complete Yogi breathing
consisting of three parts: 'abdominal', 'middle', and 'upper',
breathing.

ABDOMINAL BREATHING

Execution.—Standing, sitting or lying. Our consciousness is   Fig. 6
directed to the region of the navel. With the exhalation we draw
in the abdominal wall. Then, through the nose we *breathe in*
slowly while relaxing the diaphragm; the abdominal wall is
arched outward, and the lower part of the lungs thus fills up
with air. *Exhalation*: the abdominal wall is drawn in tightly,
forcing the air out of the lungs through the nose.   In abdominal
breathing, only the lower lobes of the lungs are filled with air
and thus only our abdomen executes a wave-like movement,
while the *chest remains motionless.*

Therapeutic effect.—A magnificent relaxation for the heart.
Reduces high blood pressure, stimulates digestion, regulates
intestinal activity. Abdominal breathing gives a splendid internal
massage to all organs of the abdomen.

115

MIDDLE BREATHING

Fig. 7   *Execution.*—Standing, sitting or lying. Our consciousness is directed to the ribs. After exhaling, we *inhale* slowly, through the nose while expanding our ribs to both sides. In *exhaling*—we contract the ribs, thus forcing the air out through the nose. In middle breathing the middle part of our lung is filled with air, while *the abdomen and shoulders remain motionless.*

Therapeutic effect.—Takes the pressure off the heart; freshens the blood circulation to the liver, gall, stomach, spleen and kidneys.

UPPER BREATHING

Fig. 8   *Execution.*—Standing, sitting or lying. We direct our consciousness to the top of the lungs. After exhaling, we *breathe in* through slowly lifting the collar bone and the shoulders, letting air flow in through the nose and fill the upper part of the lungs. In *exhaling*—we slowly lower the shoulders and press the air out of the lungs through the nose. In upper breathing the *abdomen and the middle part of the chest remain motionless.*

Therapeutic effect.—Strengthens the hilar lymph nodes in the lungs; thoroughly airs the tips of the lungs.

1. COMPLETE YOGI BREATHING

Volumes could be written about the therapeutic effects of complete Yogi breathing. Through the lungs and circulation of the blood, it fills the whole body with fresh oxygen and prana. It would be pointless to list all our organs, from the brain right down to the toes, and explain in detail how and why each is strengthened, rejuvenated and toned up through this exercise. There is not a single part of the body, not even the smallest, which is not benefited by this breathing. The salutary effect even reaches our mind, in that our entire being is filled with new strength. The mind gains peace, self-confidence and assurance. The Yogi breathing eliminates the impurities from our blood, increases our resistance, stimulates the metabolism and has a particularly great regenerating effect on the endocrine glands. This rejuvenates the entire organism. It is a frequent occurrence in Yoga schools that pupils who are no longer among the youngest, after exercising one or two months, joyously report

116

the disappearance of certain symptoms such as recession of the gums, incipient hypermetrophia, etc., which they had regarded as signs of old age and which they had not mentioned previously because they did not expect any improvement.

In India as well as at several university clinics in Europe, reputable physicians are experimenting with the rhythmic full breathing of the Yogi. In all fields of research they have achieved amazing results, particularly in cases of high blood pressure and heart disorders. The physicians in charge of these experiments have been astounded at the results attained. In numerous cases of heart disorders which had been regarded as incurable, a complete cure was achieved; in other cases when complete healing did not take place, there was at least a permanent improvement. Merely through Yogi breathing, diseased and enlarged hearts returned to approximately their original shape.

In most cases, heart trouble is merely the result of functional disturbances of other organs, most often the thyroid and the kidneys. There are excellent medicaments for the heart—digitalis, for example. While it is true that such medicines affect the heart, *they do not cure the cause of the disturbance.* Complete Yogi breathing applied in connection with appropriate mental treatment and body postures, heals the organic disturbances which have caused the heart trouble, and as a result, the heart also returns to health. Consequently, the effect of complete Yogi breathing surpasses that of any remedy which only treats the heart, even though the medicament may be one of the best there is. Specialization has caused medical science to be divided up, and therapeutics has become only an art of treating the symptoms. People forget that *the human body is an indivisible unit,* so that an insignificant little gland is often responsible for a disorder appearing in a remote part of the body.

If we have a disorder in the gall, the lungs or another organ, every part of our body, from the brain to the last pigment cell in the skin, is changed, i.e., different from the same organ in a healthy person. There is no such thing as a disease of just *one organ*: it is possible, however, for a general condition of disease to *culminate* in one organ. Thus the whole human being is sick, not just one part of his body. I was surprised for example, to find that a patient being treated for high blood pressure and

117

heart trouble had to submit to the most widely differing remedies such as bloodletting, chemical medicaments, etc., but without any success. Even the most famous professor had not thought of examining the patient's feet and his walk. This patient was suffering from a neglected case of flat feet. As a result, the *static loads on his entire skeleton were so badly disturbed that the nerves emanating from his spine became disordered* and his heart, completely unable to cope with the excessive burden caused by the improper distribution of weight, also became affected. This caused high blood pressure and degeneration of the heart. Yoga exercises restored the ankle bones to their proper position. The skeleton again carried the weight of the body in the normal manner, the dissipation of energy ceased, the backbone returned to its normal position, the nerves recovered, the blood pressure declined, and the heart, now freed from its excessive burden, quickly returned to normal.

I could cite innumerable similar cases of so-called 'miraculous' healing produced by Hatha Yoga. Actually, however, these are not miraculous, but quite natural. Hatha Yoga does not heal with chemicals, but with the forces of nature. Nature is universal, synthetic, and *man is a child of nature who cannot be divided, and specialized to pieces.*

One who thinks logically can now clearly understand the following: if Yoga exercises, and first of all Yogi breathing, have such a great healing power, how much more effect they must have on a person who has a healthy mind and a healthy body, and *always breathes in the Yogi manner*! Certainly such a person is thoroughly healthy. He is immune to all disease; he can cope with all life's difficulties and be a blessing for himself and his surroundings!

Complete Yogi breathing is the basis of all further exercises in the regulation of breath. The exercises in the following pages are only extensions and variations in this method of breathing. The *beneficial effect of complete Yogi breathing is inestimable.* Actually it should not be merely an exercise which we perform only at certain times, but rather our constant method and manner of breathing. It has no disadvantages, only advantages, and is therefore equally beneficial for those who are healthy and those who are sick. *It should be used constantly by both. Once we*

118

get accustomed to breathing in this way, we acquire a deep-seated peace of mind and such perfect self-discipline that nothing can make us lose control of ourselves. (See theoretical part).

Execution.—Standing, sitting or lying. By means of our consciousness we animate our entire trunk always following the wave-like movement of our inhalation and exhalation. In this way we experience complete equilibrium. After exhaling, we slowly *breathe in* through the nose, counting up to eight, and combining lower, middle and upper breathing in a wave-like movement (Puraka). First, we expand our abdomen, then our ribs, and finally we raise the collar bone. At this point our abdominal wall is already drawing in slightly and we begin the exhalation (Rechaka) in the same manner as the inhalation, that is, by first drawing in the abdominal wall, then contracting the ribs, and finally lowering the shoulders, while we let the air out through the nose. In complete Yogi breathing, the entire breathing mechanism, i.e., the lower, middle and upper lobes of the lungs are in uniform movement. Between the inhalation and the exhalation we can retain our breath for as long as is comfortable.

Therapeutic effect.—We experience a great feeling of peace. This exercise completely airs the lungs, increases the oxygen and prana supply in the blood, sets up an equilibrium between the positive and negative currents, calms the entire nervous system, regulates and slows the activity of the heart, reduces high blood pressure, and stimulates digestion.

Psychic effect.—The calming of the nervous system affects our mental condition. We are filled with a feeling of peace, quiet and security.

2. KUMBHAKA

Execution.—Standing, sitting, or lying. The consciousness is concentrated on the *heart*. Kumbhaka is actually nothing other than complete Yogi breathing extended through the retention of the breath. We inhale through the nose during eight counts as in the case of complete Yogi breathing (abdominal, middle and upper breathing), retain the breath for eight to thirty-two seconds (beginning with eight seconds, we add one second each day until reaching thirty-two seconds without effort). No one

119

should hold his breath longer than thirty-two seconds unless his heart is in perfect condition. If, while we gradually increase the rhythm of this breathing, we feel any strain on our heart, we must stop at the number of seconds which we can reach without exerting our strength. We exhale through the nose while counting up to eight seconds just as in the case of full Yogi breathing.

Therapeutic effect.—Balances the positive and negative currents, has a splendid calming effect on the nervous system, slows down the heart activity, and consciously regulates the pulse in case the latter is irregular. Kumbhaka is the most effective exercise to discipline the nervous system and make it conscious.

Psychic effect.—Develops the will power and determination.

3. UJJAYI

Execution.—Standing, sitting or lying. The consciousness is directed toward the thyroid gland. We *inhale* through the nose as for the complete Yogi breathing, counting to eight; then *retain the breath* (Kumbhaka) during eight pulse beats. *Exhalation.*—As in the full Yogi breathing but while counting to sixteen and expelling the breath through the mouth, we make a long drawn out 'S' sound until the air has been completely expelled from the lungs. Then we immediately begin the next inhalation and continue the cycle.

Therapeutic effect.— Through the induction of a strong positive current, the endocrine glands are greatly stimulated. This exercise has a particularly powerful effect on underactive thyroid glands, and thus increases the function of comprehension. Abnormally low blood pressure is raised. Excitable persons who have a tendency to excessive thyroid activity or excessively high blood pressure should *not* practise this exercise.

Psychic effect.—Increases mental alertness and concentration.

4. KAPALABHATI

Execution.—Standing or sitting. The consciousness is concentrated in the inside of the nose, and we pay special attention to the cleanliness of the air passages. Like all exercises in pranayama, this one begins with an exhalation. However, since the entire rhythm is brought into play through the exhalation and the main emphasis is thus placed on Rechaka, we do not exhale by a slow contraction of the abdominal muscles, but by tensing them suddenly and quickly, so that the air is expelled through the nostrils in a loud blast as if from a bellows. After this rapid exhalation, we do not pause even a second, but let our abdominal muscles relax, which, almost of itself, slowly fills the lower and middle part of the lungs with air. It is immaterial whether the upper part is filled or not, as this exercise is actually a pranayama of the diaphragm. These rapid bellows-like exhalations must be made in quick succession through a vigorous tensing of the abdominal muscles; inhaling should be made very slowly.

Therapeutic effect.—Kapalabhati is one of the most excellent exercises of the lungs. It simultaneously cleanses and tones up the nasal passages, strengthens the salivary glands and expels bacteria which have gained access to the inner nose. Through constant practice of Kapalabhati, people who occasionally relapse into the unhealthy and very dangerous habit of mouth breathing, develop into nose breathers. A further therapeutic property of Kapalabhati is that after three to five repetitions, the body is vitalized, and the solar plexus is strengthened and recharged with vital energy.

Psychic effect.—Increases the ability to concentrate.

Variation.—Kapalabhati via each nostril separately. Setting the index finger of the right hand in the centre of the forehead and holding the left nostril closed with our middle finger, we execute Kapalabhati by expelling a blast of air through the right nostril. The inhalation is always through both nostrils. Then, closing the right nostril with our thumb, we execute Kapalabhati through the left nostril. Kapalabhati, executed alternately through the left and right nostrils, is of great benefit when the air passages of the two nostrils are not equally clean.

5. SUKH PURVAK
Comfortable Pranayama

Execution.—In Padmasana ('Lotus Seat'), we place the right index finger on the centre of the forehead between our two eyebrows. After a vigorous exhalation we hold the right nostril closed with our right thumb, *inhaling* through the left nostril during four pulse beats. After *retaining the breath* during

121

sixteen beats, we release the right nostril, place the middle finger on the left nostril and *exhale* through the right nostril during eight beats. The fingers remain as they are. After *inhaling* through the right nostril during four beats and *retaining* the breath sixteen beats, we close the right nostril and exhale through the left during eight beats. Then, with the fingers remaining as they are, we repeat by inhaling through the left nostril during four beats, retaining the breath sixteen beats, exhaling through the right nostril during eight beats, and so on.

Therapeutic effect.—Positive and negative currents are brought into a powerful equilibrium. This exercise should be performed very consciously and never repeated more than three times! Persons with weak lungs should perform the exercise in a rhythm of 8-8-8 instead of 4-16-8 given above, or practise the exercise to a count of eight beats without retention of breath.

Psychic effect.—Extraordinarily strong. The mental functions and our alertness are greatly increased. One of the most important exercises to facilitate mental Yoga (Raja Yoga) in order to reach the condition of trance.

6. BHASTRIKA

Bhastrika means bellows, the movement of the lungs being compared to that of the blacksmith's bellows.

Execution.—Sitting in Padmasana or Sidhasana, we powerfully and quickly inhale and exhale ten times, after which we breathe in deeply, retaining the breath from 7 to 14 seconds. Exhale slowly. Repeat three times. We must perform this exercise cautiously, instinctively stopping at the least sign of exertion. Going to extremes can be harmful, but if not overdone, this is one of the most purifying exercises. There is a modification of Bhastrika in which only one nostril is employed.

Therapeutic effect.—A very powerful exercise, Bhastrika must not be exaggerated. It relieves inflammation of the nose and throat during chronic colds, destroys phlegm, and when mildly employed can cure asthma. It is good against cold feet, especially in winter, as it not only increases the gastric fire, but also the general warmth of the body.

Certain of these exercises are modified for the benefit of European Yoga pupils.

7. CLEANSING BREATHING

Execution.—Standing with legs apart, we *inhale* slowly through the nose as in complete Yogi breathing. When the lung has been completely filled with fresh air, the *exhalation* is immediately begun as follows: the lips are pressed close to the teeth while we keep a narrow slit open between them. Through this narrow slit we force the air out in a number of short, detached movements. We must feel as if our mouth were not open at all, and that a great effort on the part of our abdominal, diaphragmic and rib muscles is required to force the air through the small opening. If we merely blow the air out weakly and softly, the exercise is of no benefit.

Therapeutic effect.—The toxins in the blood are expelled, chronic diseases are overcome, and our immunity is fortified. The impure air inhaled in badly aired rooms—cinema, theatre or railway carriages—is cleaned out of the lungs and blood. Headaches, colds and influenza are quickly cured. In time of epidemics this exercise is indispensable, as it prevents infection. At such times it is recommended to perform the exercise five times daily, repeating it three times each time it is practised. In cases of gas or other poisonings, this breathing is a blessing.

Psychic effect.—Increases confidence, overcomes hypochondria.

8. BREATHING TO STRENGTHEN THE NERVES

Execution.—Standing with feet apart and after exhaling, we *inhale slowly*, at the same time raising both arms in front of us, palms upward, until level with our shoulders. Then we double up our fists and, while still holding the breath, draw them back quickly to the shoulders, extend the arms again, draw them back again quickly, and repeat this movement once more. While exhaling, we relax our arms, letting them sink and rest while we bend over forward. The exercise is beneficial if, when we push our arms forward, we do so as if they were being resisted by a strong force which we were obliged to overcome. Each time we must push our arms forward slowly and with a great effort so that they actually tremble with exertion. For persons who find it difficult to do this three times while holding the breath, the exercise should be repeated only twice.

123

Therapeutic effect.—Increases the resistance of the nervous system. A good remedy against nervous trembling of the hands and head.

Psychic effect.—Gives us self assurance in meeting others and increases our mental powers. We feel equal to any struggle.

9. 'HA' BREATHING, STANDING

Execution.—Standing, with feet apart, we inhale as in complete Yogi breathing. During inhalation, we raise our arms slowly vertically over the head, *hold our breath* a few seconds, then suddenly bending forward, we let our arms hang down in front while simultaneously exhaling through the mouth and pronouncing the sound 'Ha'. In *exhaling*, the 'Ha' sound is made by the rush of air itself, not by the throat. *Inhaling* slowly, we straighten up, raising our arms again vertically over our head, then exhale slowly through the nose while lowering the arms.

Therapeutic effect.—Freshens the blood circulation, thoroughly cleanses the breathing organs, combats the tendency to feel cold.

Psychic effect.—We feel cleansed. When we are in cheap tawdry surroundings, the unclean atmosphere clings to us and, even when we have left the area, causes a depression and mental nausea. In such cases the 'Ha' breathing effectively purges us from the mental poisons and quickly dispels our depressed feeling. *For policemen, detectives, specialists, treating neuralgic or neurotic patients, and others whose occupation brings them into contact with the mentally deranged or persons of low character, this exercise is a blessing as it preserves their mental health and enables them to resist outside influences.*

10. 'HA' BREATHING, LYING

Execution.—Lying flat on our back, we *inhale*, as in full Yogi breathing, simultaneously raising the arms slowly until they reach the floor behind our head. For a few seconds we *retain the breath*, then quickly raise our legs, suddenly flex our knees, put the arms about them, press our thighs to our abdomen and simultaneously *breathe out* through the mouth with the 'Ha' breathing. After reposing a few seconds, we begin breathing in slowly, raising our arms over our head. At the same time we stretch our legs upward and slowly lower them to the floor; then after a few seconds' pause, we slowly exhale through the nose while lowering the arms to the side of the trunk. Then we relax completely.

Therapeutic effect.—Similar to that of 'Ha' breathing, standing.

11. SEVEN LITTLE PRANAYAMA-EXERCISES

1.

Execution.—Standing with feet apart, we raise our arms while slowly breathing in, until the palms of the hands are touching each other above the head. We hold our breath for seven to twelve seconds and then slowly lower the arms, palms down, while exhaling. We conclude the exercise with the cleansing breathing.

2.

Execution.—Standing with feet apart, we inhale as in full Yogi breathing, arms forward, level with the shoulders, palms of the hands downward. While retaining the breath we swing our arms rapidly and rhythmically back and outward as far as possible horizontally, then forward again and backward again from three to five times; then exhale vigorously through the mouth while slowly lowering the arms; and conclude the exercise with the cleansing breathing.

3.

Execution.—Standing with feet apart. During slow inhaling as in full Yogi breathing, we raise our arms forwards until shoulder height, with palms in. While *retaining the breath* we briskly swing our arms like a windmill upward, backward and around again, three times; then do the same in the opposite direction, i.e., down, back, up, and around. *Exhalation.*— Vigorously through the mouth, while the arms are lowered. Exercise is concluded with the cleansing breathing.

4.

Execution.—Lying on the floor, face down, we put the palms

125

of our hands on the floor under the shoulders, fingers forward. After a full inhalation we retain the breath and do a slow push-up, holding the body stiff so that it rests only on the toes and two hands. Slowly we lower the body to the floor again and repeat the movement three to five times. *Exhalation.*—Vigorously through the mouth. The exercise is concluded with the cleansing breathing.

5.

Execution.—We stand erect, facing a wall, and put the palms of the hands on the wall at shoulder height, arms outstretched. After a full *Yogi inhalation*, we retain the breath and lean forward, holding our body stiff, and bending the elbows until the forehead touches the wall; then by exerting our full strength, we push our body, still holding it stiff, until it is vertical and erect again. We repeat this three to five times, then *exhale* vigorously through the mouth. The exercise is concluded with the cleansing breathing.

6.

Execution.—We stand upright, straight as an arrow, feet apart, and hands on hips. After a full Yogi inhalation, we *hold the breath briefly*, then bend forward slowly, breathing out through the nose as we bend. While slowly *breathing in*, we straighten up again; then after a short *retention* of the breath, we *breathe out* while bending backward. While breathing in again, we straighten up; then do the same while bending to the right and straightening up again. While breathing out, we bend to the left, then straighten up while breathing in. Then after a short *retention* of breath, we breathe out calmly through the nose while lowering the arms. The exercise is concluded with the cleansing breathing.

7.

Execution.—Standing erect with feet apart or sitting in the Padmasana posture, we make a full *Yogi inhalation*, but instead of drawing in the air in one movement, we inhale in short, detached puffs as if we were sniffing some odour until the lungs are completely full. We *retain* the breath seven to twelve seconds,

126

then *breathe out* through the nose calmly and slowly. The exercise is concluded with the cleansing breathing.

*   *   *

There are countless variations of the breathing exercises, but for persons who wish to practise Hatha Yoga for their health's sake, it is fully sufficient to practice those given here, alternating according to the tables at the end of this book. The other exercises are for those whose one purpose in life is to become a Hatha Yogi. Such persons, however, must absolutely have a guru (master) to aid and advise them in their practice and check their mistakes. In this book I have introduced exercises which can be practised without danger even by beginners. Those who get beyond this stage will, in any case, be drawn to the master they need. The same applies to the asanas. Even for Hatha Yogis who have reached the highest stage, the exercises given here are the most important basic everyday ones to practise. The countless other exercises which we cannot include here through lack of space, are used to develop abilities in which people of the Occident are generally not interested. On the other hand, persons who *do* have a desire to develop such abilities, will surely find the guide and master they need; for 'when the chela is ready, the guru is there'.

XIV
— — — —

Asanas
BODY POSTURES

THE proper exercise of Yoga asanas is inseparably linked with our mental experience, the guiding of consciousness, and properly applied breathing exercises. If we follow the directions strictly, we will achieve a worthwhile result; but if we practise haphazardly, breathing irregularly and without inner concentration, we cannot expect any success. Although on the one hand Hatha Yoga exercises have a physiological effect, their main aim is to take advantage of the *reciprocal relationship between the body and mind.* In order to increase the mental effect, it is recommended that most exercises be performed with the eyes closed.

Hatha Yoga exercises should be done on a hard floor, not on a soft sofa or mattress. Indians exercise on a small rug or mat which is never used by anyone else. They begin their exercises with meditation.

1. PADMASANA
Lotus Seat

Figs. 9, 10   *Execution.*—Sitting on the floor, we put the right foot on the left thigh and the left foot over the right one on to the right thigh. The farther back we bring *the foot towards the abdomen, the easier this exercise is to do!* The lotus flower in India is the symbol of mental purity and the completely developed consciousness. Just as the lotus, in its spotless, snowwhite, untouched purity, floats over the waters of the swamp, so the pure mind of the Yogi soars, untouched by carnal desires, over the temptations of lower physical instincts. This posture is comparable to the

128

complete equilibrium and isolation of the lotus flower. The complete symmetry of our body increases the harmony of the distribution of power. This posture preserves the equilibrium of our positive and negative currents and heightens the effect of breathing exercises. Padmasana is the most suitable posture for the breathing exercises which are performed sitting. We hold our consciousness in the heart; breathing regularly and sitting immobile, we do not allow our thoughts to run freely, but force them to obey our will. In this way we consciously store up a tremendous amount of creative energy. The effect is comparable to that of a great river which is suddenly dammed up. In the rising waters lies tremendous power. Precisely in apparent inactivity and in disciplining his thoughts, the Yogi controls and retains the out-flowing creative energy. Through not thinking, not speaking, and not acting, a powerful positive force is stored up.

Therapeutic effect.—Mental and physical stability and general calming of the nervous system. The effect varies depending on the breathing exercises with which the lotus seat is combined.

2. SIDHASANA
Posture for Meditation

Execution.—We sit on the floor, cross our legs, tailor fashion, then place the right foot on the left thigh. Persons who find Padmasana too difficult should practise Sidhasana. This posture is suitable for meditation.

Therapeutic effect.—The same as that of Padmasana.

3. YOGA-MUDRA

'Mudra' is Sanskrit for 'symbol', 'example'. This exercise is a symbol of Yoga! In performing it we experience impersonality. *Figs. 11, 12, 13*

·*Execution.*—We sit in the lotus seat with our legs crossed, or we sit on our heels. In the lotus seat, we press our two heels against the lower part of the abdomen, then inhale in the Yogi manner. We breathe out, while bending slowly forward until our head touches the floor, putting our arms behind our back and clasping our left fingers about our right wrist. In this position we remain as long as we can without breathing; then, while

129

slowly breathing in, we gradually straighten up and end the exercise with a slow exhalation.

Therapeutic effect.—This exercise restores order among the organs of the abdominal cavity which have slipped from their position as a result of colonic inertia or degeneration of the stomach and intestinal nerves. The regenerative effect is brought about by external and internal muscular massage and intra-abdominal pressure. Yoga-Mudra develops powerful abdominal muscles and strengthens the loins. The mental effect is very great. This exercise is extraordinarily beneficial to persons who are inclined to be proud. Pride is driven from us. We learn to bow humbly before God and to turn to the source of life within us.

4. SUPTA-VAJRASANA

Figs. 14, 15

Execution.—We assume this posture by first kneeling on the floor with our feet apart, lowering our body until we are sitting on the floor between our heels; then with the aid of arms and elbows we lower the trunk until the back of our head touches the floor. We place our hands behind our neck. We breathe without effort and remain in this position as long as we can do so without feeling undue strain. We guide our consciousness to the solar plexus and the region of the heart.

Therapeutic effect.—This exercise causes a general tension in the legs, particularly in the knees and thighs, and also has a stimulating effect on the nerves beneath the skin. Tiny blood vessels are freshened and the activity of the pores is particularly intensified. Through the sharp bending of arms and legs, the blood circulation is retarded in the limbs and blood is forced into the trunk to the main nerve centre in the solar plexus. This is a highly stimulating and regenerating exercise of excellent effect for people with a dull nervous system and underactive glandular functions. Hypersensitive people should practise this exercise only for a very short time and very cautiously.

5. ARDHA-MATSYENDRASANA

This exercise is unique in its kind. It is probably the only one in the world which strengthens the backbone through a twisting movement to the right and to the left. It is named for the Yogi Bagavan Matsyendra. However, since the original exercise is very difficult, it has been included in Hatha Yoga under the name of 'Ardha'(semi)-Matsyendrasana. This exercise also causes difficulties for beginners for a certain time. For this reason Srimat Kuvalayananda, Director of the Lonavla Research Laboratory, prescribes a simplified version known as Vakrasana 'twisted posture', which has almost the same effect. Let us first consider the Ardha-Matsyendrasana exercise.

Execution.—We place the right heel under the left thigh. The Figs. 16, 17 right leg rests horizontally on the floor. Now we put the left foot over the right thigh, setting the sole of the foot on the floor. The chest is turned to the left, the right arm is put in front of the left knee standing vertically, and with our right hand we grasp the left ankle. Then we slowly twist the back to the left, turning our head in the same direction. With the left arm we reach backward and with the left hand we grasp the left knee. (See picture). We guide our consciousness into the spine, and although the lungs are pressed together, we breathe with an even rhythm. We remain in this position until we instinctively feel that we have had enough. Then we change feet and legs and execute the exercise in the opposite direction.

Therapeutic effect.—As already mentioned, we can only keep our backbone in perfect health if it is exercised in every possible direction. The backbone can be bent in six directions: forward, backward, right and left with twists to the right and left. By Sarvangasana, Halasana, Paschimotana, and Yoga-Mudra, the backbone is strengthened through forward bending. Matsyasana, Bhujangasana, Salabhasana, and Dhanurasana strengthen it through flexing it backward. Ardha-Matsyendrasana or Vakrasana is the only exercise which twists the backbone to the right and left.

This asana overcomes spinal deformities and has a beneficial effect on the entire nervous system, the liver, pancreas, spleen, intestines, and kidneys. Together with Bhujangasana, this posture can be considered as a preserver of the kidneys. The blood supply to the vertebrae and to the nerves branching out from the backbone is increased to the maximum and, in this way, exercises a therapeutic and rejuvenating effect on the entire organism. One of the most useful exercises!

An easier modification of this asana is shown in Fig. 16.

131

In this posture the spine is held upright without any twist. We use complete Yogi breathing. Consciousness is held in the spine.

Therapeutic effect.—Self-confidence, determination, and perseverance.

6. VAKRASANA I AND II
Twisting Posture

Fig. 19   *Variation I.—Execution.*—We sit on the floor with our legs stretched out in front of us. Drawing the right leg towards us so that the thigh and the knee are pressed hard against the abdomen and the chest, we lift the right foot over the left and place the sole of the right foot next to the left thigh on the floor. The palms of both hands are placed flat on the floor, fingers outward. The consciousness is led into the backbone, and we experience equilibrium and self-confidence. After three full Yogi breathings, we change feet and repeat.

Therapeutic effect.—The positive and negative currents are brought into equilibrium.

Variation II.—Execution.—The posture is the same as that for Variation I, that is, the right leg drawn in and put over the left. The entire backbone including the head is turned as far as possible to the right. The right arm is stretched out behind the back, and we put the left arm in front of the right knee such that the left armpit presses the right knee backward. We concentrate on the backbone. After three full Yogi breathings we change feet and repeat.

Therapeutic effect.—The same as Ardha-Matsyendrasana but Fig. 18   milder. For a further variant see Fig. 18.

7. MATSYASANA
Fish Posture

Fig. 20   *Execution.*—Starting in the Padmasana posture, with the help of our elbows we lower the trunk backward until, with our chest arching upwards, the top of our head is resting on the floor. The hands grasp the toes. We breathe lightly and avoid even the slightest tension. The consciousness is directed towards the thyroid.

Therapeutic effect.—Overcomes any stiffness in the **neck**, while the tension in the opposite direction brings all muscles of the neck into play. The muscles of the back are contracted, and the chest and abdominal muscles are tensed, making it possible to breathe regularly during the exercise. The backward pressure of the head causes a brisk flow of blood to all the organs of the neck. The blood flowing out of the heart meets strong hindrances, collects in the neck and thoroughly cleanses the thyroid, the tonsils and the adenoids. This exercise is excellent for colds and purulent tonsils.

8. PASCHIMOTANA

Execution.—Lying on our back on the floor, we raise the arms, Fig 21
while inhaling deeply, until the arms are flat on the floor behind us. Then, while breathing out calmly, we sit up slowly, bending forward, until our fingers touch our toes or until we can grasp our ankles. The knees must remain completely stiff. The head is bent forward until it touches the knees, and our elbows rest on the floor. While breathing in deeply again, we sit up and lie back slowly on the floor, our arms at rest next to the body. Exhale and relax. The consciousness is held in the solar plexus.

Therapeutic effect.—This exercise is excellent for the abdominal organs and is only equalled in its effectiveness by Halasana. The major and minor Psoas, the *Quadratus Lumborum*, the lateral abdominal muscles and the recti are strengthened in an extraordinarily effective manner by this posture, as they are completely contracted and remain so during the entire asana. This exercise has a very powerful effect on the nerves of the small of the back. The functions of the organs of the lower extremities, the loins, and the pelvis are controlled by the Lumbo Sacralis nerve centres and two minor *plexi*. Paschimotana stretches and strengthens these nerves. Simultaneously, functional disturbances of the stomach, liver, spleen, kidneys, and the intestines are prevented. As a remedy for constipation and intestinal catarrh, this exercise is invaluable. Loss of appetite and underactivity of the liver and kidneys are cured. According to the experiences of physicians in the Yoga research institutes in India, haemorrhoids and diabetes have been checked in their development and even healed. The exercise when repeated serves as a very effective means of reducing fat around the abdomen. The efforts called for by the lateral muscles develop well proportioned, slender hips. The *sexual organs*, rectum, prostate, uterus and bladder, together with their nerves, are abundantly supplied with blood, and their condition is very much improved. The backbone is made more pliable. Beginners, particularly men, find this posture difficult. With diligent practice, however, even the stiffest spine becomes elastic. Thanks to the magnificent exercise of the abdominal muscles, Paschimotana is rightly called the 'source of vital energy'—by the Yogis.

9. PADAHASTASANA
Stork Posture

Fig. 22 *Execution.*—Exactly the same as Paschimotana, but standing.

Therapeutic effect.—The same as that of Paschimotana, but here the blood is forced to the head in a stronger stream and therefore the effect on the brain is intensified.

10. UDDIYANA-BANDHA
Drawing in the Abdomen

Figs. 23, 24, 25 Uddiyana means 'upward flight', 'upward climb'; Bandha means 'drawing together' or 'blocking'.

Execution.—Standing with feet apart, trunk bent slightly forward, we hold the arms straight and place the hands upon the slightly bent knees. After a full Yogi inhalation, we slowly exhale and draw the abdominal wall in tight by raising the diaphragm as high as possible just as if our internal organs had disappeared. This 'sucking in' of the abdomen can be even better achieved if we arch in the small of the back and press with both hands on the knees. In this position the rectus muscles of the abdomen relax as if the abdomen were being pushed in by compressed air. With diligent practice we become more and more expert at 'drawing in' our abdomen. It is not an easy matter, as the muscles functioning in this exercise are ordinarily independent of our voluntary control and must now be made 'conscious'. With the necessary concentration, however, we can do it. This type of asana is to be performed only with an empty stomach.—One of the most excellent exercises!

Therapeutic effect—Almost every asana is more or less an exercise to overcome colonic inertia. Let us not forget that most cases of lazy colon result from chronic catarrh of the large intestine. The two asanas which India has given to the Occident as a sovereign remedy for this fashionable disease of civilization are Uddiyana and Nauli. In these exercises, the large intestine and the diaphragm together with the appendix, are lifted. The contents of the intestines are compressed, peristaltic action begins, and the waste matter collected in the convolutions of the colon is set in motion. The nerves which govern intestinal movements, are practically 're-born' after the Uddiyana exercise. This exercise is also an excellent remedy against prolapses of the stomach, intestines, uterus, etc.

Uddiyana can also be practised in Padmasana.

11. NAULI

This asana is just the opposite of *Uddiyana-Bandha*. It could also be called a central isolation of the rectus abdominal muscle. It has four variants: Nauli-Madyama, the central isolation of the *rectus abdominis*; Dakshina-Nauli, isolation of the rectus on the right side; Vaman-Nauli, isolation of the rectus on the left side; and finally, Nauli-Kriya, twisting of the rectus abdominis. *(Figs. 26, 27, 28, 29)*

Nauli is one of the most difficult exercises, because in this movement the rectus abdominis and the other muscles are pushed forward while contracted so that they form a ridge in front of the abdomen. In this exercise, too, these muscles must be made responsive to our voluntary control.

Execution.—We stand in the same position as for Uddiyana. We breathe out vigorously and perform Uddiyana. At the same time we contract the abdominal muscles—the two recti—and arch them forward with a strong push. When isolating the right or the left rectus, we bend to the right or the left. Through the pressure of our hands on our knees we can assist in isolating these muscles. As variants, Dakshina-Nauli and Vaman-Nauli may be executed in the same manner as ordinary Nauli except that an alternating pressure is applied by the hands on the knees. When the rectus muscle is to be drawn to the right (Dakashina-Nauli), the right hand is pressed more firmly on to the right knee, while the left hand is relaxed. Vice-versa for Vaman-Nauli. Nauli can be learnt in several weeks, while in other cases several months may be necessary for its mastery. With diligent persistence and close observation of the abdominal muscles, we can learn this exercise even without a teacher. The fourth variant of Nauli, the rotation of the muscles, is the most difficult. It is achieved through executing a long slow circle with the hips—like the 'Hula-Hula' dancers in Hawaii—then transmitting this rhythmical circular movement to the isolated abdominal recti muscles. This exercise is also practised without breath after an exhalation, and after finishing it, we inhale vigorously.

Therapeutic effect.—Similar to that of Uddiyana-Bandha, but the deep-seated muscles of the back which hold the abdominal muscles in place are strengthened and regenerated by an abundant flow of blood. All organs of the abdominal cavity receive automatic massage, their activity is stimulated and brought into equilibrium. Uddiyana and Nauli, when exercised alternatingly, stretch the spinal column, particularly in the lumbar region. In addition to their other advantages, both exercises are a great help for those who concentrate their entire energy on mental development and for this reason lead a life of continence, as these exercises prevent nocturnal emissions of semen.

12. TRIKONASANA
Triangle Posture

Fig. 30   *Execution.*—Standing with feet apart, we raise the arms sidewards, palms upward, as far as shoulder height. Throughout the exercise we hold our arms out in a straight line with the shoulders. While raising our arms to this position, we make a full Yogi inhalation. While exhaling, we bend the trunk to the right until we touch the right toes with the fingers of the right hand. In this position we stretch our arms vertically and turn our face upward. As we straighten up, we inhale and then, with only a moment's pause, we slowly bend to the left and exhale. After a short pause, we straighten up again as we inhale, then slowly lower the arms sidewards while breathing out. The consciousness is held in the spine.

Therapeutic effect.—This movement gives lateral exercise to the backbone. The lateral muscles of the trunk are alternately flexed and relaxed. The trunk is flexed to the right and the left, and all the dorsal muscles which hold the vertebrae come into play. The lateral muscles and the backbone are animated. The vertebrae are subjected to lateral compression and tension.

136

The backbone is made resilient, and the bones and muscles of the hips are put in order. After infectious diseases, this exercise accelerates complete healing, as it aids in dissolving the toxic accumulations in the organism. Numerous latent infections are expelled from the body.

13. BHUJANGASANA
Cobra Posture

Bhujanga means 'cobra'. This asana was so named because it gives the body a similarity to the cobra with its head raised. Fig. 31

Execution.—Lying face down on the floor, we put both hands, palms down, on the floor below the shoulders. With a full Yogi inhalation, we slowly raise our head as far as possible. Then by tensing the muscles of the back, we lift our shoulders and trunk higher and higher and farther backward without helping with our arms. The arms are only used to prevent us from sinking back on to the floor. While performing this exercise, we feel how the pressure on the vertebrae in our neck gradually spreads lower and lower down the spine. In the last phase we can also use our arms to help bend our trunk backward. However, we must pay attention to keeping the navel region near the floor. After remaining in this position and holding our breath from seven to twelve seconds, we breathe out slowly as we gradually return to the prone position. During the exercise, we first hold our consciousness in the thyroid, and then, as our backbone is flexed more and more, our consciousness shifts lower and lower until it finally reaches the lower part of the spine near the kidneys. As a variant the consciousness can also be guided into the entire spine.

Therapeutic effect.—While we remain in the cobra posture, the intra-abdominal pressure increases, and the two recti muscles of the abdomen are tensed. As a result of the abundant flow of blood to the backbone and the sympathetic nerves, the entire abdomen and the trunk are regenerated. Gradually, through diligent practise, we overcome the stiffness of the backbone and any deformities which it may have. This exercise also has a highly beneficial effect on the deeper lying abdominal and back muscles. Every vertebra, ligament, and tendon is tensed and forced to work. When we remember that thirty-one pairs of nerves leave the spinal column and that the two main cords of the sympathetic nervous system are embedded in the muscles on both sides of the backbone, we can easily understand the beneficial effect this posture has on the entire nervous system.

The kidneys, too, are regenerated and given an abundant supply of blood. In India this asana is used chiefly to prevent calculus formations in the kidneys. During the exercise, the blood is squeezed out of the kidneys, but as soon as the body returns to its original position, a vigorous flow of blood invades them and washes away any deposits. The thyroid glands are stimulated and any functional disturbances are corrected. Persons suffering from excessive thyroid growth should not practise this exercise!

Bhujangasana, like the other Yoga asanas, differs from occidental sports in that we must remain for a length of time in the tensed position. This is precisely the secret of the beneficial effect. This exercise is also useful in developing self-confidence and overcoming inferiority complexes.

14. ARDHA-BHUJANGASANA

Fig. 32

Execution.—We kneel on the left knee, putting our right foot forward, so that the shin is vertical. We make a full Yogi inhalation. While exhaling, we shift our weight from the left knee to the right foot, slowly lowering the trunk until our hands, hanging downward, touch the floor. The backbone must be held upright. We remain thus from three to seven seconds without breathing and then slowly rise again during a full Yogi inhalation. We repeat this three times and then change feet.

Fig. 33

Here is another variant: Just as in the first exercise, but during the shifting of the body weight on to the right foot, we twist the body to the left, also turning our head to the left; with our arms somewhat spread, our palms forward, we touch the floor with our fingers. After repeating this three times, we change feet and do the turn to the right.

Therapeutic effect.—The resilience and elasticity of the entire bone structure is preserved and improved. Fatty deposits about the hips are prevented, and our feeling of equilibrium is enhanced.

138

15. SALABHASANA
Grasshopper Posture

Salabha is Sanskrit for 'grasshopper'. In this posture we raise Fig 34 the legs like a grasshopper; hence the name.

Execution.—Lying face down, with the nose and forehead touching the floor, we place our fists on the floor beside our thighs. We make a full inhalation, retain the breath, and by pushing our fists against the floor, we raise our outstretched legs as high as possible. After remaining thus for a few moments, we return to the original position and exhale. This exercise requires a great effort but its effect is astonishing. The consciousness is held in the pelvis and the lower vertebrae.

Therapeutic effect.—A result of our unnatural way of living is that a high percentage of modern mankind suffers from constipation. Our sedentary way of living weakens the intestinal walls, as the insufficiency of exercise causes inadequate blood circulation and prevents the nerves in the intestines from fulfilling their stimulating function. The great majority of Yoga asanas has a beneficial effect on the activity of the intestines; and among these postures, Salabhasana is one of the most effective. By providing a powerful stimulus to the internal organs, it puts an end to even the most persistent case of constipation. The concentrated tensing of the muscles affects the digestive glands, located along the digestive tract and increases the supply of blood to the mucous membranes.

This posture tenses all the extensor muscles, while the flexors relax; the pressure in the abdominal cavity increases and the nerves in the region of the small of the back, the loins, and the lower vertebrae are strengthened. This exercise is one of the most excellent movements for the muscles of the back. The other effects are the same as those of Bhujangasana, especially with regard to cleansing and rejuvenating the kidneys.

16. ARDHA-SALABHASANA

Execution.—Just as for Salabhasana, except that we raise one Fig. 35 leg and then the other instead of both together.

Therapeutic effect.—The same as that of Salabhasana, but less intense. This exercise requires much less exertion.

17. DHANURASANA

Bow Posture

Fig. 36 *Dhanur* is Sanskrit for 'bow'.

Execution.—Lying on the floor, face down, we inhale slowly, reach back, and grasp both ankles, arching our back and remain-in this posture as long as possible. During this exercise we breathe slowly and hold our consciousness in the pelvic region.

Therapeutic effect.—This exercise has a highly stimulating effect on the endocrine glands. Starting with the thyroid, it affects the thymus, hilum, liver, kidneys, superenal capsule, pancreas, and especially the sexual glands, strengthening them and increasing their activity. This exercise is very beneficial in cases of underactive thyroid and is likewise effective in stimulating the other endocrines. It is thus helpful in cases of diabetes, and incipient impotence, sterility, etc. In both men and women the symptoms of sexual weakness characteristic of the climacteric are postponed for a long time, and youth thus preserved into old age. Children who are slow of comprehension should practise this daily, as the constant stimulation of the thyroid aids the latter's development, thus improving the activity of the brain. For women this exercise is excellent in cases of disturbances and irregularities of the menses. The entire spinal column and all nerve centres are strengthened, and their resilience preserved. Both the stimulating effect on glandular activity and the tensing and contraction of the muscles tend to prevent accumulations of fat. This exercise is thus the best remedy for morbid obesity! The effect of the exercise can be heightened if we rock gently to and fro during the posture. In the beginning it is probably fatiguing as the backbone is not so flexible, but with diligent practice, we become more and more adept. For persons with a sedentary way of living, this exercise is a blessing, as it banishes fatigue pains. Dhanurasana should *not* be performed in cases of hyper-function of the thyroid or excessive growth of any of the other ductless glands. The exercise should be begun very cautiously, and only little by little should we increase the length of time we hold the posture. The solar plexus is recharged with vital force.

18. MAYURASANA
Peacock Posture

In Sanskrit the word 'Mayura' is approximately equivalent Figs. 37, 38 to 'peacock'. This asana is called 'peacock posture' because it reminds us of a peacock spreading its tail.

Execution.—We kneel down, on the floor, knees apart, palms down on the floor, fingers toward our feet, as we squat on our heels. In this position our elbows come to rest under our abdomen. Bending forward we touch the floor with our forehead which balances us as we raise our feet and stretch our legs out behind us. Then we raise our head, so that we are supported only by both arms. This exercise is one of the most difficult asanas and requires long practice.

Therapeutic effect.—An excellent exercise for equilibrium. The control of positive and negative energies must be supported by mental concentration. The stunted nerves of the lower trunk and the abdominal cavity are regenerated, colonic and general intestinal activity is stimulated, and constipation cured. This is one of the exercises which increases intra-abdominal pressure. Its therapeutic effect is therefore very great for the organs of the abdominal cavity. Through the pressure of the elbows on the abdomen, the flow of blood through the descending aorta is retarded, while as soon as the pressure is removed at the end of the exercise, the flow of fresh blood flushes the digestive organs. In this way, and through the increase in pressure in the abdominal cavity, the digestive organs are cleansed and regenerated. Another important therapeutic effect of this exercise is its great influence on the pancreas gland. It is thus a means of preventing or curing diabetes.

19. SARVANGASANA
Pan-physical Pose or Candle Posture

In Sanskrit 'sarva' means 'whole', 'entire', while 'anga' means 'body'. Sarvangasana is thus the 'asana of the entire body'. This posture consists of four parts and belongs to the most important asanas. It is of such a great benefit to the entire organism that everyone should practise this exercise several times daily. Its extraordinarily wholesome effect is partially due

141

to the fact that in this posture *we receive opposite currents*. It is well known that the earth emits *negative* currents, while we receive *positive* currents from universal space. In our normal upright posture, we thus receive negative currents through our feet and positive ones through our head. In the next three exercises, Sarvangasana, Viparita-Karani and Sirshasana, the effect is the opposite. The fact that the entire organism is upside down is the cause of their great therapeutic value. The effect of these exercises is much greater than that of short waves and other ray treatments.

Figs. 39, 40   *Execution.*—Lying on our back, with our arms extended next to the body, palms on the floor, we slowly inhale and lift our extended legs without bending the knees until our legs are vertically *above us*. As soon as we reach this position, we raise the trunk so that our hips rest upon our hands. From here we push our trunk upward until it and our legs are in a straight line vertically above us. Our chin is pressed firmly against our chest. We breathe abdominally and remain in this posture as long as we feel it is comfortable without exertion. Beginners should only remain in this posture briefly and gradually increase the time. To conclude the exercise, we slowly lower the trunk and then our feet to the floor. Never drop down like a sack!— Then we remain for a few seconds, breathing smoothly, uniformly, in order to allow the blood circulation to return to its normal channels. *Don't jump up suddenly!* This is very injurious for the heart. As we can see, the most important asana, Sarvangasana, is so simple that it can be performed by any child. *Two months' practice of this exercise are of much greater benefit to the circulation, the metabolism, and our mental alertness than the most expensive medicaments or a holiday trip.*

Therapeutic effect.—Regarding the physiological effect of Yoga asanas, the reader has already been able to form an opinion from the results achieved by the Yoga research institutes in India, so that with regard to Sarvangasana, the reader can himself understand the excellent therapeutic effect.

In order to assess properly the inestimable effect of Sarvangasana, let us consider the influence of the posture on the body itself. Sarvangasana, as mentioned above, primarily gives us the terrestrial radiations in a direction opposite to the normal one. While in this position the force of gravity also has a reversed effect upon us. Those organs which in normal life are in the upper part of the body and therefore receive a smaller flow of blood (as the heart must overcome the force of gravity in order to pump the blood to the head and the organs in the neck region) are now below. This means that the blood pours into these organs of its own weight without the least exertion on the part of the heart. Thus the burden on the heart is reduced, and as long as we remain in the Sarvangasana posture, the heart gets a rest, initially brief and later increasing gradually in duration. This relaxation for the heart is even more beneficial than that obtained while we are lying down.

At the same time the lungs and all organs about the region of the neck are flushed and cleansed by a fresh flow of blood. By pressing our chin against our chest, we prevent an excessive rush of blood to the head and by means of abdominal breathing, we press the veins together so as to avoid congestion. The veins of the neck are nevertheless filled with blood so that the thyroid, tonsils, ear glands, hilum, thymus, and the lungs receive fresh nourishment. For this reason, Sarvangasana is the most effective therapeutic and rejuvenating remedy for these organs. Bhujang-asana and Dhanurasana have a great stimulating effect on the thyroid. Sarvangasana, Virparita-Karani, and Sirshasana, on the other hand, not only calm and strengthen the thyroid, but also the other organs mentioned above. These exercises are thus the complements of the stimulating exercises.

The thyroid is the organ responsible for our sense of time. Thus the thyroid determines whether we move, speak, perceive, and comprehend quickly, or whether we perform all these functions slowly. Persons with an underactive thyroid gland cannot keep up with their fellow men. They are always coming in late, as their feeling for time is inadequate. Their heart beat, intestinal activity, and other vital functions are slow. On the other hand, people with excessive thyroid function are always in a hurry, breathe hastily; their pulse is too quick, their intestinal activity forced, and their manner of speaking is often an incomprehensible chatter. These irregularities are adjusted and normalized by the exercise of the three inverted physical postures which have a tonic effect on this extremely important

143

organ. The organs of the abdomen which, owing to gravity, are normally supplied with an abundance of blood—because the blood in flowing downwards expands the blood vessels—are held above the other organs when we practise Sarvangasana. These abdominal organs are thus relieved of the excess of blood. The blood vessels contract again and recover their resilience. From medical experiments we know that the system of blood vessels has an astonishing capacity for regeneration. Persons suffering from varicose veins find that the exercise of Sarvangasana or the other two inverted asanas—even if practised for only a few minutes a day—has a miraculous effect on haemorrhoids and difficult cases of varicose veins. Morbidly distended veins flatten out, and their walls contract to normal dimensions. Even the worst cases of varicose veins can be cured if we practise this exercise three times daily. People whose profession requires a great deal of standing, such as dentists, sculptors, carpenters, waiters, etc., can prevent distension of the veins if they practise the above-mentioned asana several times daily, particularly after work.

For women, Sarvangasana banishes the ever present menace of irritation and catarrh of the uterus. Excessive quantities of sluggishly circulating blood are diverted and the lower abdominal organs are thus calmed and relaxed. These exercises are a great aid to juveniles during puberty as well as to all persons wishing to live a continent life. The undesirable abundance of blood is led off from the sexual organs, the blood is distributed in a beneficial manner to the chest and the organs of the neck, and the individual's thoughts and desires are diverted from erotic channels. The danger of nocturnal emissions which menaces boys during puberty is completely banished if these exercises are practised before going to bed. During sleep, the superfluous blood, drained out of the parts of the body where it is not desired, is led towards the head and thus is able to promote a development of mental faculties.

If we want our children to enjoy an excellent growth mentally and in every other respect, we should see that they practise Sarvangasana, Viparita-Karani or Sirshasana at least three times daily, morning, noon and evening. Their growth is largely regulated by the thymus gland, and these three above-mentioned

144

exercises of Hatha Yoga also have a magnificent influence on this gland. Adults should practise these exercises in order to maintain their health, their youthful vigour, and resilience until advanced old age. For *old age* does not necessarily mean bodily decay and decrepitude. A practical example for this is given by the Indian Hatha Yogis and the many students of the Occident, who, after demonstrating in practice the beneficial effect of Hatha Yoga, preserve the perfection of their body until far into old age.

Sarvangasana has no disadvantageous effects. Long lost youth, vital force, and once-dissipated energy stream back abundantly even into the bodies of elderly people who all feel as if they were newly born. The functioning of the ductless glands which have become disordered as a result of inadequate thyroid activity, returns to normal, and the organism which has begun to struggle against incipient diseases obtains new strength. Sarvangasana is the most perfect rejuvenating and relaxing exercise for the nerves.

20. VIPARITA-KARANI

Viparita in Sanskrit means '*inverted*', while *Karani* means Fig. 41 '*effect*'. The name of this asana thus points out three things: 1. the fact, mentioned in the discussion of the asana above, that we receive radiations from the earth and from cosmic space in an inverted position; 2. the posture of the body; and 3. the reversal of time. When standing on our feet, we grow old whereas in the *Viparita-Karani posture*, we become younger!

Execution.—Lying on our back, we slowly inhale, raise our legs upward and, supporting our hips with our hands, gradually raise our trunk until it is resting on our shoulder-blades. Our legs and feet are inclined slightly beyond our head, and precisely this is the difference between Viparita-Karani and Sarvangasana. Another difference is that our hands support our hips, not our trunk. By slow abdominal breathing we prevent an excessive inflow of blood. We remain in this posture as long as it is comfortable without exertion. In between times we exercise Jivabandha three to four times. (See Simhasana.) We then slowly return to our prone position on our back; then relax and calm ourselves by Yogi breathing before standing up.

145

Therapeutic effect.—Very similar to that of Sarvangasana. In India this exercise is used effectively to cure goitre, Basedow's disease and even feeblemindedness in children. Diseases of the breathing organs are avoided if we practise systematically. Incipient colds or tonsilitis are cured in many cases, or the disease is made to run its course faster. This is a favourite exercise of women, as it smoothes away or prevents wrinkles in the face. Viparita-Karani causes a flow of blood to the skin and muscles of the face which is of more value than any kind of massage or electric treatment! (See also the therapeutic effect of Sarvangasana.)

21. SIRSHASANA

Figs. 42, 43, 44, 45, 46, 47, 48

This posture is the third most important asana. 'Sirsh' in Sanskrit means 'head', and we can thus speak of this as the Yogi head stand.

Execution.—We kneel, interlace our fingers and put our hands before us on the floor. Leaning forward, we place the head on the floor with our interlaced fingers supporting the back of the head. With the help of our feet we raise our hips up in the air. Then we also lift our feet and bend our knees until we are in equilibrium standing on our head. By slowly straightening the legs, we bring the entire body into a straight vertical line. In this position we remain as long as we can do so without effort. Our breathing is calm and slow. To come down from this position, we first bend at the hips and the knees until we reach a kneeling position on the floor. In this position we assume a resting pose by placing the fists one over the other on the floor and the forehead on top of the upper fist. It is important that we do not suddenly fall over, as such a shock can nullify the benefits of the exercise. For the same reason, once we have reached the resting pose, on the floor, we should not suddenly jump up again, but remain in this position for a few seconds in order to allow the circulation of the blood to return to its normal channels.

Therapeutic effect.—This asana differs from the two previous asanas in that the emphasis here is on the brain which is supplied with blood and prana.

The most important organ of our earthly existence is the brain.

146

It is the permanent seat of our consciousness and a mighty power house upon whose perfect functioning all our manifestations and our value as human beings depend. And yet how little attention we pay to it! Let us remember that our intellectual faculties, sight, hearing, the functioning of our other organs of sense, the amazing split-second precision of our entire nervous system, proper movement of the limbs, the power of our sexual organs—hence even the attributes of our future children—all this depends on the quality of the nervous centres in our head! This magnificent gift of God deserves to be better cared for.

Of all the asanas Sirshasana is the exercise which for children, assures the perfect development of the brain, and for adults, the maintenance of mental health.

During our normal activities, the heart has to work hard to overcome the pull of gravity in pumping blood up to the head. By merely lying down, we make its work much easier. Here too, however, civilization has spoiled man and led him away from the ancient natural way of living. Civilized man sleeps with his head atop a pile of pillows, thus preventing his neglected brain from receiving the rich flow of blood it so urgently needs. Most of the nervous disorders which plague our civilized world are caused by inadequate nourishment of the brain. *At first we feel easily fatigued; later our memory begins to fail; our head and hands begin to tremble; and our sight, hearing, and other organs of sense become dull and unreliable. This is followed by disturbances of the sense of balance, vasomotor disorders, neurasthenia, hysteria, melancholy, depressions, claustrophobia and other phobias and a thousand other conditions which all originate in the neglected condition of our brain.*

And then comes the 'miracle'! After much persuasion the neurasthenic begins sceptically and indifferently to practise 'Sirshasana'. In his first attempt he does not succeed in standing on his head and is only able to lift his hips; his feet seem as heavy as if they were nailed to the floor. But nevertheless somehow or other he already feels better. He feels refreshed. 'Coincidence!' he tells himself. The next day he tries it again, at first against the wall, and this time manages to raise his legs off the floor. He still cannot get them up straight, even though he tries and paws the ground like a balky mule!—Finally he gives

147

up, gets to his feet again, and . . . what a wonderful sensation he feels! He laughs! . . . And quickly tries it again. . . But his legs still refuse to obey. He looks in his book and reads, 'The beginner should not practise Sirshasana more than three times in succession'. 'Too bad!' he says and can scarcely wait for the next day. Again he has made progress! He is almost able to stand on his head properly! And so day by day with increasing diligence he practises until some evening he succeeds in standing on his head for a few seconds! The next day this person who so far suffered from inferiority complexes, suddenly turns into a show-off. Boasting of his ability, he stands on his head and demonstrates 'Sirshasana' to his colleagues at the office in the morning and to his family or friends in the afternoon. His success is capital. He is admired and envied. Proudly he goes home and settles down comfortably in an easy chair to read his paper. He starts to reach for the glasses he has worn ever since his eyes started to 'play tricks' on him. But suddenly he notices that he can even read the smallest letters without difficulty. He cannot believe his eyes, turns and twists the paper back and forth, and finally has to admit joyfully that he could 'see pretty well' up to now, but his arms 'were probably a bit too short'. Now, however, he sees splendidly and can read the finest print without any effort and without glasses. Suddenly he realizes that for a number of days he has not heard the usual buzzing in his ears and that other neurasthenic symptoms have disappeared. Last night he was so sleepy that he forgot to take his usual sleeping tablets, yet he slept soundly till morning.

This is no exaggeration! Even the first attempt at Sirshasana brings an abundant flow of blood to the brain, the eyes, ears, nose, mouth, the tonsils, adenoids, thyroid, lung tips, etc. The heart is relieved of a great part of its burden and filled with new energy. . .! All the splendid results which have been achieved through the practice of Sirshasana cannot be listed. Countless Yogi pupils, rejuvenated or youthful, who have recovered their strength to work again, as well as persons in middle or advanced age who have suffered from the most serious symptoms of neurasthenia, can prove that the Hatha Yoga exercises—primarily Sirshasana—have a magnificent therapeutic effect.

However, we must correct an erroneous belief which keeps

148

numerous elderly people from practising the inverted exercises.
'I cannot do a head stand; I might burst a blood vessel in my
brain!' they say. Don't believe it! There is no experience of any
kind to back up this baseless fear; one may have a stroke lying,
standing, walking or in any other position of the body, not because the individual was precisely in that position, but rather
because there were already serious disorders in his organism, in
the distribution of positive and negative currents, production
of hormones, and in other vital functions. Numerous elderly
pupils practise regularly in the Yoga research institutes in India.
I myself, in my Yoga school, have observed very many elderly
Yoga pupils who practised Sirshasana every day. One of them
was a man of over eighty. But in no case has there ever been the
slightest disadvantageous effect. On the contrary, the results
have been excellent. Most of the great Yogis are unbelievably
old by European standards but none of them would ever think
of avoiding the inverted asanas 'because a blood vessel in the
head might burst'. I have only heard this idea in the Occident
where people have strayed far away from mother nature. To
cite another example, Indians frequently practise an exercise
involving concentration on the point of the nose. In this exercise
one looks at the point of the nose with both eyes. People in
India practise this exercise without a second thought, and no
one has ever had his eye 'get stuck'; on the contrary, the
muscles of the eye are strengthened and made more alive by this
exercise. In Europe people are afraid of such a thing, and tell
children 'don't look cross-eyed—your eye might get stuck!' I
have asked many people whether they had ever seen anyone
whose eye had taken on a squint because of looking cross-eyed.
'No', they said, 'but people say so'. And so it is with the head
stand and the blood vessel which might burst in the brain.
No one has ever seen a person get a stroke and fall over because
of standing on his head.

But one thing is certain: persons suffering from high blood
pressure *must not perform asanas in inverted positions*. First of
all they must bring their blood pressure back to normal through
pranayama exercises and other asanas. As soon as the high
blood pressure has returned to normal, we can begin with the
three most useful asanas. I thus repeat what I have said in the

previous chapter: An ailing person should not practise Yoga without a competent instructor. *The healthy persons can do it without any hesitation at all.*

Finally we must not neglect to mention that these three inverted exercises, in addition to their miraculous effect on the health, have a further advantage which makes them rate as important exercises among Indian Yogis.

Occidental medical science has confirmed that our brain contains nerve centres which are not used by people of average development. In such persons these nerve centres are lying dormant, and medical science has not as yet discovered their purposes. These centres are very well known to Indian Yogis, as the latter have found out through thousands of years of research how to waken and activate them. All exercises of Hatha Yoga, particularly Sarvangasana, Viparita-Karani and Sirshasana, whether we wish it or not, tend to awaken these centres and give us possession of faculties which are generally unknown. Ordinarily, people do not even believe that such faculties can be achieved.

Such faculties include telepathic communication, clairvoyance, viewing the past and future, and other so-called occult powers. These latter are attainable by anyone who seriously practises Hatha Yoga. One who doubts this can convince himself as soon as he has taken the time and patience to develop his nerve centres beyond the stage reached by the average man! In this connection see also the therapeutic effect of Sarvangasana. Yogis call this the 'King of all the asanas'.

22. HALASANA

Figs. 49, 50, 51

This asana is called 'plough posture' as it resembles the Indian plough. 'Hala' is Sanskrit for plough.

Execution.—Lying on our back with out-stretched arms, palms down, beside the thighs, we exhale slowly and lift both feet just as in Viparita-Karani, but carry our feet on beyond our head until our toes touch the floor. Our arms remain flat on the floor, palms down. This is the first phase of Halasana. In the beginning, we remain in this posture from ten to fifteen seconds while breathing slowly and regularly. The second phase is more difficult. Whereas in the first exercise we put our toes on the floor, quite near our head, this time we push our feet much

150

farther backwards. We breathe deeply and must constantly pay attention to keeping our knees stiff. In this second phase our weight shifts more toward the top of the spine. In the third phase, our weight is supported by the vertebrae of the neck, so that our entire spine takes part in this exercise. In the third phase we push our feet—knees still stiff!—still farther behind us, draw in our arms and clasp both hands behind the neck. We remain in this position a few seconds, as long as possible without exertion, and then slowly 'unroll' until our feet return to our starting position.

Therapeutic effect.—Among the various asanas, Bhujangasana, Dhanurasana and Salabhasana subject the outside of the spine to compression and the inside to tension. Halasana and Paschimotana do just the opposite, putting compression on the inside and tension on the outside. These exercises have a beneficial effect on all the vertebrae, as in their various phases every part of the spinal column is subjected to compression or tension. In this manner the blood circulation is thoroughly freshened, and a fresh blood supply is assured to the most important nerve centres along the vertebrae. That is the explanation for the amazing effect of Halasana. We can banish fatigue or exhaustion instantly through Halasana. We immediately feel refreshed and in full possession of our strength again. This splendid exercise not only benefits the nerves of the spinal column but also the vertebrae themselves. Persons whose vertebrae have been pulled out of position through a sedentary way of life can restore their spine to normal by means of this posture. Children with spinal deformities can be brought back to normal in an almost miraculous manner. Body symmetry is enhanced to the point of perfection, and simultaneously the production of negative and positive currents is balanced. The tensing and flexing of the back muscles has a regenerating and strengthening effect on them. The organs of the abdominal cavity are tightly compressed and their blood supply increased. This exercise has a rejuvenating effect on the sexual glands, the pancreas, liver, spleen, kidneys, and suprarenal glands. Experience has shown that Halasana has excellent results in cases of disorders of the menses, and in difficult cases of diabetes is has often brought about a complete cure without any insulin treatment.

Fatty deposits are prevented and accumulations of fat around the abdomen and the hips disappear completely; hence actors, actresses and others who must pay attention to their figures can preserve their youthful shape through daily exercise. This asana also has a strengthening effect on the organs of the thorax and the region of the neck. The entire glandular system including the glands of the brain is rejuvenated thanks to the reciprocal relationships existing among these glands. Halasana stimulates brain activity and heals the disorders which have been caused by anaemia of the brain. Headaches frequently disappear immediately. Halasana is one of the best exercises to develop the spine and the nerves of the back. If we remember that young people have a flexible spine, whereas a stiff back is generally one of the characteristics of old age, we can immediately understand the excellent effect of this asana.

People with an excessively stiff backbone should be cautious when beginning this exercise. We should bend backwards slowly and cautiously, not all at once, in order for our muscles to meet the unusual demand without too much exertion and without damage. With a few weeks' diligent practice, even the stiffest spine begins to limber up.

23. BRU-MADYA-DRISHTI
(Fixation between the eyebrows)
NASAGRA-DRISHTI
(Fixation of the Nose Tip)
SWINGING THE EYES
ROLLING THE EYES

Here are four excellent eye exercises to preserve normal vision and to develop the faculty of concentration.

The first exercise is performed as follows. Sitting in the Padmasana posture we inhale deeply, then breathe regularly and look at a spot between the eyebrows, i.e., we direct the eyes towards a spot above the bridge of the nose. If we feel the slightest fatigue, we pause and rest for a moment, then repeat the exercise, but this time look at the tip of the nose. In this posture we remain breathing regularly until we feel fatigue. Then we exhale and rest.

Immediately after this exercise it is good to perform two

further exercises which strengthen the eyes in a most extraordinary manner and which, if practised daily, help preserve the
youthful fresh resilience of the eyes until a ripe old age. These
movements are *swinging and rolling the eyes.*

Eye swinging is performed as follows: In the Padmasana
posture, we first look straight ahead. Then while inhaling deeply,
we turn our eyes to the right as far as possible. While slowly
exhaling, we then return our eyes to looking straight ahead.
Next, while breathing in deeply and slowly, we turn our eyes to
the left as far as possible; then, slowly exhaling, we bring them
back to the centre. This is repeated three times.

Eye rolling is executed as follows. First we look straight
ahead; then while exhaling, we look downward. Now while
slowly inhaling, we start to describe a circle with our eyes to the
right and upward until they have reached the top centre. At
this point we begin to exhale and continue rolling the eyes
towards the left and downward until we reach the bottom centre
again. Here we begin again with the inhalation and continue
to the right and upward until we have completed the circle
three times. Then after a short rest we begin the roll in the
opposite direction. After a few weeks of such exercise, weak eyes
are regenerated. Persons who practise these excellent exercises
from their youth onward need not wear glasses until far on into
old age!

It is highly important that we perform these exercises *consciously* with our *full attention and concentration*, and very slowly.
Only in this way are they of real benefit.

24. SIMHASANA
Lion Pose

Hatha Yoga does not neglect a single important muscle of the
body. Why, therefore, should we forget the tongue, whose
peculiar movements immunize us against numerous diseases
of the throat! Simhasana is practised in Padmasana posture or
Sidhasana, and during this movement we breathe regularly.

Execution.—We arch the tongue back, exerting pressure with
the tip of the tongue on the palate; now we bend our head
forward, touching the chest with our chin and extending the
tongue as far as possible. Then we draw our tongue back,

153

pushing the tip hard against the palate again. This stretching out and drawing in of the tongue is repeated ten to twelve times, and each time the tongue is arched upward against the palate.

Therapeutic effect.—The civilized Occidental, once he has outgrown his childhood, never 'sticks out' his tongue again, except when his doctor asks him to say 'ah'. This is a great mistake! Just as merely walking around is not sufficient for the muscles of the thigh and calf, if we want to remain perfectly healthy, our tongue, too, needs more exercise than it gets through speaking and the little work involved in chewing. As has been shown by the research work of Srimad Kovalayananda in Lonavla, Simhasana has the following therapeutic effect: The good exercise of the neck muscles immediately improves their blood supply. The nerves and glands of the neck become healthier. The throat and larynx get a special massage. The thyroid and its auxiliary glands are strengthened. The hearing is improved, the secretion of saliva becomes more complete. The throat is cleansed and incipient tonsilitis is cured.

Jiva-Bandha, or 'tongue-block' is the name of the first phase of Simhasana, where the tongue is arched upward and pressed against the palate. This exercise is combined with that of Viparita-Karani. (See Viparita-Karani).

25. SAVASANA
Corpse posture

Fig. 66   'Sava' in Sanskrit means 'corpse'. This asana is called the 'corpse posture' as it is the last and serves for rest and relaxation after the other exercises.

Execution.—We lie on our back, with both arms extended near our body. Our feet are together and our legs likewise stretched out to their full length. Without exertion we slow down our breathing as much as possible. We rest. Beginning with our feet, we relax all our muscles. One after the other, we concentrate on the muscles of the entire body, the feet, shins, knees, thighs, abdomen, arms, shoulders, neck, and head; then we consciously leave them so that all are completely relaxed and remain so. The entire body is so relaxed that we do not feel it. We withdraw our consciousness to the heart and experience only the deepest rest and peace which brings perfect health.

154

Therapeutic effect.—The nervous system gets complete rest. This is the most perfect exercise for relaxation, for we should realize that *the relaxation of the muscles is just as important for their development as their activity*! The circulation of the blood is now in complete equilibrium, and its distribution is regular. The circulation in the veins becomes easier; high blood pressure declines rapidly. The heart is relieved, as its work of pumping is made many times easier. Ten minutes' rest in this posture, with our breathing slowed down and our thoughts concentrated on entire and perfect rest, is more valuable than a full night's sleep. Savasana could also be called *'active passivity'*, as we consciously and intentionally withdraw ourselves from all parts of the body into the heart and achieve the same conditions as in sleep—except that we are awake.

*   *   *

This posture ends the list of asanas. The Yogis recommend that they be practised daily, whether we are young or old, man or woman. Before I begin to list the Yoga exercises to be performed daily, let us consider for a moment what people of the Occident, in their high-speed living, have not yet learnt; namely, what it means to *rest* in the Indian sense of the word!

Our body is a factory equipped with machines. The wastes, toxins, and products of oxidation are 'swept out' of our organism during sleep, just as in a factory, when the machines are standing still after hours, the time has come for cleaning and repairs.

In addition to the regeneration of sleep, however, civilized people should re-learn the long-lost art of relaxing the way primitive people and animals rest. This perfect form of rest is called 'muscle relaxation' in Hatha Yoga. If we lift a dog or cat when it is resting, we notice that its whole body is as limp as a rag. Its muscles are soft and as relaxed as a lump of dough. This is what the Yogi means by 'rest'!

As a rule occidentals are even in a hurry when they have nothing to do and when—in their opinion—they are resting. Even when they are lying down and apparently resting somewhat, their muscles are at least half tensed. The current of prana and flow of regenerating forces within the organism, however,

155

does not begin until we are at complete rest for a few minutes. In the Lonavla laboratory recent experiments have proven that a quarter of an hour of perfect Yogi rest cleanses the blood of dangerous toxins.

In the morning before we get up and at night before we go to sleep we should practise this relaxing, resting posture. Even during the day we can very often find an opportunity. Not only among the orientals who are capable of resting for hours in apparent inactivity, but also among Europeans, there are exceptional persons who, amidst the hustle and bustle of life, even in a pause between two business transactions, are able to drop all their affairs and problems and, in any desired position, give themselves over to complete rest.

It is a long established rule that everyone should have holidays every year. Everyone should be able to spend at least a month in complete physical and mental relaxation in order to store up enough energy and vitality for the next year. But let us look at how much rest and relaxation the occidental actually gets. The majority of Europeans and Americans really begin to get nervous when their summer vacation starts. First they have to decide where they are going! Then come feverish preparations, packing, disputes with porters, renting a car, etc., and above all, the excitement preceding the journey. In a fashionable bathing resort, the unlucky guest has everything but rest. Our gregarious instincts come to the forefront. The resort hotel even provides entertainment, and out of courtesy every self-respecting lady and gentleman comes down to five o'clock tea and to the evening entertainment. The next day the same guests tire themselves out with excursions or at the beach, as they are not accustomed to such physical exertion; and in the evening there is dancing again. Then there are others who are already playing bridge half an hour after their arrival. Instead of enjoying the mountain sunshine or the ozone-laden sea air, they stay in the same tobacco smoke as at home. Instead of being relaxed and rested, their nerves are 'calmed' by strong coffee and even stronger alcohol! Sleeping is limited to only a few hours! The next day they go out into the hot sun with an over-exerted heart! Thus most people come home from their holidays and return to their daily work, brown but exhausted.

156

This is no summer vacation, much less relaxation! This is the surest way to exhaust our motor prematurely. The organism which has already become susceptible to disorders and whose vitality is lowered because of our inappropriate way of living, will not be able to fight off the diseases and other dangers which lurk at every turn. A small percentage of western sports fans who do not particularly care for summer-time amusements and social gatherings, fall into the opposite extreme. These people belong to the group of passionate hikers and boaters who carry their tent and kit for hundreds of miles uphill, down-hill and over high mountain ranges in order to reach the summit. Such sporting exertions practised under the pretext of 'summer-time fresh air' can later lead to enlargement of the heart valves and other disorders.

Let us go to the beach of a great city! Among the bathers there are very few who withdraw to the quiet of a remote spot, to lie on the soft sand, close their eyes, think of nothing, and deliver themselves up to the sheer blessed delight of perfect relaxation. No! Most city dwellers go to the beach in groups; or they go there to meet their own circle of friends. The older people sit in the warm water and chat for hours, and the young ones play, primp, and flirt on the beach or in the water. All of this goes on in the torrid heat of sunshine, as these people have no real idea of the physiological effect of the sun's rays. They do not know that sunshine is only a powerful therapeutic agent when taken in small doses. If we get more sunshine than our nervous system can stand, it is a deadly poison! But vanity demands that we have a becoming tan! Poor little nervous restless chocolate-brown people—even smoking cigarettes at the beach!—you should know that a half day in the hot sun at the beginning of the summer season is as hard on your heart as if a new untrained cyclist were to pedal a bicycle for fifty miles. If only you knew what damage is done to your *endocrine glandular system*, expecially the *thyroid*, by an overdose of sunshine!

The seashores of India—where it is not much hotter than central Europe in the dog days—are not alive with bathers until towards the evening, as these people know from experience that bathing and swimming are most beneficial in the evening. During the day under the blazing sunshine, one may also take a sunbath, but never longer than ten minutes. Only when our skin has begun to tan can this length of time be extended by a few minutes. The Indians with their naturally brown skin are in a more favourable situation in this respect than the white-skinned occidentals. But even so, Indians do not spend hours at a time in the blazing sunshine. When they want to swim, they do so in the evening after sunset. In India every child is brought up to know that all intensified body postures under the burning sunshine are damaging. Basking like a crocodile for hours at a time in the sunshine is no less so. An old Indian proverb has a symbolic meaning in this connection: 'Only a fool goes about in the sun when he can sit in the shade'. . . . In the West most people avoid the beach when the weather is cloudy or the sun is not shining brightly. They believe it is wasted effort and that the sun is 'too weak' to add anything to their tan. On the contrary, real beach-goers and true 'water lovers' know that the sun's effect is really the strongest when the sky is clouded and hazy. At such times the skin is tanned uniformly, not spottily. And when the sun *does shine* we can get a beautiful tan even by taking an air bath in the shade. Even if we swim in a shady spot, the mirroring effect of the water and the rays of the sun which filter through the clouds will give us just as good a tan as the direct sunrays would do.

We people in southern India cannot understand at all why occidentals are so desirous of having a brown skin. All southern Indians are olive brown, but this does not make them feel the slightest bit happier or more valuable than northerners who are quite fair. When I came to Europe *I was surprised to find that most people in the West want to be brown in order to show off and make others envious*! Southern Indians would never think of boasting that their skin is darker than that of their northern compatriots! What claim to fame and honours does one have by reason of being black? I have never yet found a sun-roasted, chocolate-brown European who could answer this question for me . . . .

We now come back to the question of *'right relaxation'* which we have mentioned above. Because of the intense and constant nervous strain of western life, it is not easy to learn this. Lying on our back without any heavy or constricting clothing, we let our arms lie, palms upward, at our side; we

158

relax all our muscles, and think of nothing in the world; that is, without identifying ourselves with them, we let our thoughts run freely until they tire, their running slows down, and our brain runs 'empty'. Probably everyone has experienced this peculiar condition, when the excited, restless, whipped up nervous system takes hold of our thoughts by force. During the most intensive work, we suddenly stare off into space, all of our thoughts disappear, and our brain turns into a vacuum. If some one speaks to us, we do not answer, because we do not hear or do not understand. After one or two minutes the brain 'switches itself on' again, and we slip back into our daily routine. We feel that our work, our thinking, and our general condition are better and fresher. This is nothing else than the involuntary 'switching off' of our thoughts when we are burdened by excessive mental work. It is relaxation of the mind and body for one or two minutes.

Now this refreshing rest and relaxation can be brought about under even more satisfactory conditions when we practise it four to five times daily as an exercise. Lying on our back, with our muscles relaxed, we wait until our thoughts 'run down'. Having thus 'lost ourselves', we are at rest. Our last conscious thought as we go into relaxation and our first 'animating thought' when we set our imagination into action again is that we are completely at rest, lying there with no tension, and that we want every last muscle of our body to be relaxed. If someone were to raise our hand while we are in this condition, it would drop like a lifeless rag. After resting thus, completely relaxed, for four to five minutes, we may feel that one part of our body— generally the hand or foot—jerks a bit as if by a spasm. This is a sign that we have withdrawn completely from our body, turning over its work to the regularly functioning energies of nature. Thus the disharmonies of our personal imperfect self can no longer interfere in a disturbing manner. This relaxing, liberating, resting exercise performed on our back for five, ten or fifteen minutes is called Savasana.

Whenever possible we practise this exercise out-of-doors in the forest, under trees, or on the beach, as well as in the morning and evening in bed—but not when we are propped up by pillows! If we remember the remarks about the spine in Chapter I, we will understand why it is so important for the spine to lie flat. Whenever we have a few minutes during the day—even during our working time—we can practise this exercise. We should not wait until we are almost collapsing with fatigue!

In concluding our description of Hatha Yoga, we should merely like to say that one who practises the ancient pranayama and asanas not only comes into the possession of the perfect mental and physical health but also achieves an understanding of the greatest secret in the world: MAN!

XV

——— —

The Miracle of Slow Motion
Exercises

PRIMITIVE man did not need to be taught any physical exercises.
His simple way of living and his out-door activities: hunting,
fishing, running, climbing trees, throwing stones, swimming,
fighting off wild animals, throwing spears, etc., were far better
than our modern sports and gave him the most perfect physical
exercise with the maximum concentration of his attention.
Primitive man had to be a universal genius, as he was forced to
satisfy all his needs with the sweat of his own brow and the
strength of his own two hands, according to plans devised by
his own thinking.

This meant that from dawn until late at night his day con-
consisted of constant exercise. Thus he not only remained
healthy, but his muscles also developed tremendous strength.

However, as soon as he began to become civilized, he restric-
ted himself to certain activities. He delegated to others part of
the work that he had been doing previously. And now we have
reached the unnatural situation in which part of humanity does
practically no physical work at all, while the remainder is over-
burdened with heavy, stultifying labour. If we give just a little
thought to this overspecialized condition, we immediately
recognize the underlying cause of innumerable diseases which
plague mankind because of the misuse of vital force within us
and the resulting unnatural conditions of life.

The daily routine of the occidental office worker is a crying sin
against health. Nevertheless the number of adults who feel the
need of sports and take some exercise at least every second day is
very small. It is easily understandable that in the haste and hurry

161

of modern life those of us who are not wealthy and have to earn our living by mental work scarcely have any time for sport. We live in our monotonous daily 'mental routine', without giving our body what it needs. Our entire exercise consists of a little bit of walking in conjunction with our movements between home and office—held to a strict minimum by extensive use of trams, buses, trains, the underground, and motor-cars—plus the manipulation of a knife, fork, and spoon at meal time. It is no wonder that this degenerated way of living, continued for years at a time, finally saps our vital strength to the point where it is no longer equal to the continual attacks against it. Our mental worker living in physical inertia thus falls easy prey to the most diverse diseases. It is a well-known fact that regular sports can free even the most confirmed afternoon napper from the feeling of drowsiness which he experiences after mealtimes and against which he has struggled in vain.

However, for persons who work only physically, this one-sidedness is just as disadvantageous. The mower, the factory hand, the bricklayer, all do physical work from morning until night, but they will never obtain a perfect muscular system or perfect health. Physical work can only develop the body and make it resistant when it is performed with an abundance of variations as if we were playing a game and exerting each muscle uniformly. Natural physical exercise and the instinctive longing for sporting games is part of men's heritage. While man was living under natural conditions, mother nature took care of seeing that every muscle and every part of his body was developed and strengthened. Both work and play were part of his life; but not work as performed by multitudes of working people today! This is nothing but stultifying servitude. No, in ancient times it was the highly diversified activity of primitive man, the native tribesman, soldier, and pioneer. This activity consisted of the natural movements of the body in performing hundreds of different kinds of useful acts in which the mind participated as much as the body.

All western sports are able to develop the muscles, but these sports should not be indulged in to excess. All types of sports represent an exertion for the heart. 'Athlete's heart' is a widespread and well-known menace for every sportsman. In addition, with very few exceptions, the various kinds of sports develop the muscles only in a one-sided way. The fencer develops a strong right arm and right thigh, the tennis player a strong right arm, and the skater strong thighs and calf muscles. On the other hand if we wish to develop our muscles uniformly we must practise several different kinds of sports simultaneously. But who has so much time? Now by means of the ancient Indian method for developing muscles, everyone can build a symmetrical, balanced body without expensive sporting equipment or a surplus of time. All we need is a mirror and fifteen minutes every day. With this system of slow-motion exercises, which prescribes no stultifying gymnastics but consists of movements like a game, combined with strong mental concentration, powerful muscles are developed in a very short time. Thus *everyone can indulge in sports at home*. This system gives us an excellent possibility to exercise diligently every day.

The oldest muscle-building Indian 'Dhandal and Bhasky' exercises differ from western gymnastics primarily in that they do not consist of thoughtless repetitions but of exercises performed with great interest. *While exerting our will power or imagination, we observe the moving muscles and send a flow of prana to them.*

In exercises performed consciously and purposefully, we use our faculty of imagination and conquer the inhibitions of the subconscious, our doubts and scepticism. If for example we slowly bend our right arm, constantly watch this movement, and imagine that at this very moment, a large quantity of prana is flowing into our biceps and simultaneously supplying our whole arm with blood,—we have already achieved the result! See also Chapter X—'Constructive Power of the Consciousness'. After a few weeks of diligent practice of this simple physical exercise, combined with mental concentration, we suddenly realize that our arm muscle has grown as much as if we had been doing hard work for several months. *The constructive power of consciousness will give the muscles the shape and the size which we hold in our imagination.* Let us try this method on the other parts of our body: if we use our imagination to send vital force to various parts of the body, persistently developing strength, and if we watch our muscles during our exercises or watch them in a mirror, we will soon build up a body so beautiful that even athletes will admire it.

The secret of the tremendous effect of 'slow motion exercise' on the muscles and the entire organism lies in the constructive work of the consciousness. As discussed in the chapter on the control of consciousness, the tiny nerve ends that penetrate all the tissues of the body are charged with power by the conscious will. During our exercise these tiny reservoirs are filled with a quantity of prana so that the muscles continue to build up not only during the exercises themselves but also afterwards, even during our sleep, in obedience to the dictates of our will and in filling out the forms pictured in our imagination.

Among children and even among juveniles the power of the consciousness can, within certain limits, even transform the bone structure according to the directions of the will. This can be understood by those who have not only tried it in theory but also experienced it in practice. After a short period of exercise, we can experience the constructive power of consciousness in our own body. As a result of the mental influence, these exercises, carried out with the help of auto-suggestion and concentration, are of infinitely greater benefit to the muscles and the organism than any sport performed thoughtlessly.

The Indian system of slow-motion exercises accomplishes miracles if we practise it diligently every day. No equipment is needed; for Yoga prescribes simple, natural, movements in imitation of the daily 'sports' of primitive people. As an example, let us describe the first exercise.

Fig. 67   *Javelin Throwing.*—We close our right fist as if we were grasping a spear or a javelin. Standing with legs apart and our left arm stretched sidewards, we draw back our whole body as if we were going to throw the javelin. We draw back our right arm and bend our trunk back slightly. This is the basic position. Now we go through the motions of throwing the javelin, clear to the last phase when the right hand holding the javelin is stretched out in front of us and the left arm is behind. During the movement, we flex the knees first right; then left. *We must constantly keep all our movements smooth, rhythmic, plastic, and graceful. It is very important that we perform all these exercises nude or in a bathing suit, if possible in front of a full length mirror.* When

164

exercising in a room it is very important to have a mirror, as it enables us to concentrate our thoughts on the harmony of our movements and the play of our muscles.

The actual movement is as follows: In front of the mirror we assume the basic position for javelin throwing and, tensing to the absolute ultimate every muscle involved, we go through each phase of the 'sport' as slowly as if we were watching ourselves in a slow motion film. The movement must be so slow that the exercise which, under normal circumstances would take two to three seconds, takes from thirty seconds to a full minute. By turning our head slightly to the side we can watch the movement of our muscles and our entire body in the mirror; we can see our muscles swell up as they perform the work, and with our imagination we send prana to them. After completing the movement we remain in the last phase for a full minute and then return to the basic position just as slowly. The exercise is repeated two or three times. Finally, with quick shaking movements, we relax all the muscles used. The exercise is concluded with a few deep breathings.

Many occidental sportsmen and trainers will laugh at these exercises. However, before they express an opinion, they should try out the effect of slow motion exercises *for at least a week* themselves, then they will see the astonishing results. The consciousness 'draws' or 'paints' the forms of the new powerful muscles in accordance with our desire, when we consciously send our energy to the body with our full attention. There is no lung, however weak, that will not respond to the power of consciousness and show signs of development, even in adults. Everything depends on our imagination, our will, and on whether we have faith. Everything in which we have faith succeeds. BELIEVE IN THAT WHICH IS NOT, IN ORDER THAT IT MAY BE! The imagination is the creative power in our hands.

The second exercise which should be performed daily is Fig. 68 *Shooting with Bow and Arrow.*

Standing with feet apart, we turn slightly sideward as if holding a bow in our left hand. Standing firmly, we tense the muscles of the thighs and the arms and, holding out our left arm, draw the bow string back with our right hand and then release it. The whole exercise should take approximately a

165

minute and we end it by shaking our muscles and performing several deep breathings.

Fencing.—We assume the stance of a fencer. As if holding a sabre in our hand, we spring forward and backward, dealing out blows to the left and right—but all as slow as a snail!

Weight Lifting.—We bend forward, grasp with both hands an imaginary heavy weight, and snatch it up to shoulder height. Flexing at the knees and jumping into the weight lift stance with feet apart, we then push our 'weight' up over our head with outstretched arms. Standing before the mirror and watching our movements, we perform this exercise so slowly that it takes a full minute. Finally—as ever—we shake our muscles to relax them and end by deep breathing.

Wood Chopping.—This is one of the most important primitive exercises. Standing with feet apart, we raise both arms before our mirror, imagining that between our two fists, one over the other, we are holding the handle of a heavy axe which we raise and lower as if chopping an imaginary log. We 'chop' so slowly that each stroke takes one or two minutes. Again we shake our muscles and end with deep breathing.

Fig. 69
Fig. 70
Shot-put. See illustrations.

Running.—Running is also a natural sport of primitive tribes: In front of our mirror we go through the motions of running without actually leaving the point where we stand. Breathing slowly, we consciously direct prana to all muscles involved. Again we end the exercises by shaking our muscles to relax them, then perform several deep breathings.

Boxing.—Standing before our mirror, we assume the hunched over posture of a boxer. We deal out a number of left and right jabs to an imaginary opponent; then bending over forward, we give him a few left and right body blows. Again all of this is performed as slowly as possible, with the complete concentration of all our attention and the full tensing effect of every muscle involved. End by shaking our muscles and breathing deeply.

Swimming.—This exercise corresponds to swimming training such as is given in Europe. Lying on our stomach on a narrow bench or a high stool, we go through the motions of swimming, constantly thinking of regulating our breath. Then we lie on our back and 'swim' back stroke or back crawl. The importance of

166

swimming as a natural sport has already been discussed in connection with pranayama, and we emphasize again that in addition to all other physical exercise, everyone should swim for at least half an hour daily.

Mowing.—Likewise an excellent exercise for developing back and side muscles and preserving the elasticity of the spine. The movements to the right and left stimulate the nerves branching out from the spinal column. We go through the motions of mowing to the right and to the left; then bending over forward, we 'cut' short grass with a 'sickle', likewise in slow motion. End by shaking our muscles to limber up; then several deep breathings.

Rope Climbing.—A very important body building exercise, Fig. 71 this movement can be varied in several ways. Its purpose is to imitate the natural exercise of climbing tree trunks, vines, etc. It is exceedingly simple. If exercising out of doors under the trees we grasp a thick branch overhead; at home in our room, the door frame will do. At first we hang motionless for several seconds, gradually increasing this time to several minutes. Then, after resting for a moment, we again grasp the branch or the door frame and 'chin' ourselves as many times as we can.

Crawling on All Fours.—Civilized adults may feel that this exercise is beneath their dignity. Nevertheless it is extremely beneficial. Crawling on all fours for only five minutes has the same beneficial effect on the circulation, the brain, and the endocrine glands as the asanas in inverted positions. In crawling on all fours we must naturally not slide about on our knees, but move forward with outstretched arms and legs so that our head hangs down. The physiological effects of this position have already been discussed in earlier chapters. For one or two minutes we crawl about with our arms and legs as stiff as possible; then again, but more slowly, with arms and legs bent; finally we end by crawling on our elbows. This is the so called 'Indian crawl'. When practised for several minutes, this is one of the most excellent exercises for developing the muscles.

Drawing water from a well.—Standing with legs apart before Fig. 72 our mirror and bending over forward slightly, we slowly go through the motions of pulling on a rope to hoist a heavy bucket of water out of a well. Hand over hand we reach down and grasp the 'rope', drawing it up so that when our left arm is bent with

167

our hand near our chest, our right hand is reaching downward nearly to the floor to get another purchase on the rope. Then we pull the rope up with our right hand while our left hand reaches downward. We end by shaking our muscles and doing a few Yogi breathings.

Fig. 73

Pulling a rope.—Standing with feet apart before our mirror, we reach out with the right arm, 'grasp' an imaginary rope, and pull it in with all our strength, while we turn the trunk to the right. Then with the left arm, we pull to the left. This alternating movement is one of the best exercises for the back. But here again we must not forget that the emphasis is on keeping all our movements as slow as possible in order to direct each phase with our consciousness. Our movements must be completely harmonious.

Rope Climbing.—This exercise is the same as the preceding except that our 'imaginary rope' is hanging vertically instead of horizontally. Thus we go through the motions of pulling down on it in order to 'climb' it.

Fig. 74

Wrestling.—In front of the mirror, we wrestle with an imaginary opponent. In this exercise our slow movements have a particularly graceful effect. Now and then, in between the various holds, we practise Kumbhaka. In this latter exercise, our breath should never be held for more than seven seconds.

The movements for football, ice-skating, tennis, skiing and putting the shot can also be practised in slow motion.

Why is is necessary to have a full length mirror for these slow motion exercises? This is actually a concession for the benefit of occidentals who are practising at home. Indians practise these 'Dhandal and Bhasky' exercises simultaneously with their guru (master). While concentrating, the pupils can watch the magnificent interplay of muscles in their master's beautiful, symmetrical body. They are thus practising 'according to pattern'. Their subconscious mind registers the picture of their master's perfect body which attained its beautiful build through exercises just such as these. This high degree of association and prana concentration can only be carried out when we are practising with such a perfectly developed teacher. As this is not always possible in the Occident, a mirror is an excellent substitute, although in this case we must imagine the beautiful, muscular

168

forms ourselves—without a 'pattern'. For this reason, it is helpful to hang a few pictures of well-developed athletic bodies around our mirror. If we are unable to obtain a large mirror, we can practise in the evenings in front of a lamp, watching the movements of our shadows on the wall. We must try to produce only beautiful movements as we constantly watch ourselves, either in the mirror or in our shadow.

If we have never gone in for sports, our body and our muscles represent a rough mass like the uncut stones before the sculptor. Has anyone ever seen a sculptor work on a stone with his eyes closed, checking and criticizing his work only when it is finished?

Just as the sculptor constantly watches the slow development of his work and enjoys the fact that the amorphous material is being animated through his attention while he derives faith, inspiration and strength from his work, similarly we must admire the play of our muscles, the harmonious movement of the body, and the rapid development of our muscles until the amorphous 'dead' material has turned into a living monument with athletic muscles. This unique system of ancient exercises which combines faith, will power and imagination with physical movements is worthy of serious attention and thorough study by physical training teachers in the Occident.

XVI

— — — — —

Nothing Without Mind

ALTHOUGH in this book I have only dealt with the Indian rules concerning the physical body—a discussion of the higher Yoga wisdom has been given in my book 'Yoga Uniting East and West'—Hatha Yoga is nevertheless permeated through and through with the basic elements of mental Yoga. A few words on the subject are pertinent here.

Before giving the broad outlines of the basic principles of the higher Indian philosophy, I must emphasize once more the extraordinary effect which physical exercises—performed with the co-operation of the mind—have on the muscles.

Thoughts—the manifestation of the mind—are all powerful and forge our fate for better or worse. In the chapter on the reciprocal relationship between body and mind, we learnt that with the aid of good and positive thoughts we can attract good and desirable conditions; whereas negative, bad thoughts, bad feelings propel us towards evil, misery and sickness. The force of thought dominates our earthly life, our contacts with others, our business, and our habits. The power of concentrated thought, when we know how to organize it and radiate it by means of suggestion, is so great that with its help the initiated can easily control the will of other people. The Yogi, however, does not aim at this result, but merely wants to manifest his unity with God.

The splendid scientific experiment conducted by Professor W. G. Anderson of Yale University, in connection with measurement of thought and mental power should be mentioned in this context. A student was placed on a very sensitive balance so that the centre of gravity of his body was exactly over the centre

170

of the balance. Now the professor gave the young man some arithmetic problems to do, causing an increased flow of blood to the student's brain. As a result of the change in the equilibrium of his body, the balance inclined in the direction of his head. The more difficult the arithmetic problems were, the more concentratedly the student was required to think, and the greater was the deviation from horizontal on the balance. As a continuation of the experiment, the professor asked the student to concentrate on physical exercise, think that he was performing ten to twenty deep knee bends and that his leg muscles were getting tired. After a few minutes the balance inclined in the direction of his feet—a surprising proof that the power of mind alone sufficed to direct the flow of blood towards his legs, and this purely as a result of imaginary exercises. This experiment was also carried out by Professor Anderson on several members of his audience with similar results.

In order to investigate more thoroughly the miraculous effect of mind on the body and the muscles, the professor measured the separate strength of the right and left arms of eleven of his young students. On the average, the students' right arms exerted a pull of 120 lb. Now the professor put his eleven students through a very carefully prepared, one week's 'one arm' gymnastic course. Precise measurements made at the end of this week showed the surprising fact, that while the average strength of the right arm had increased by 6.6 lb., the power in tension and thrust of the unoccupied left arm had increased during the period by an average of 7.7 lb.! This experiment proved that the brain, which was controlling the gymnastic exercises with interest, not only sent blood to the muscles being exercised, but also *strengthened and developed the inactive left arm.*

Prof. Anderson constructed a special 'see-sawing bench' which was in absolute equilibrium when he lay upon it. If he concentrated on thinking he was dancing a jig, the part of the bench under his feet began to sink. The German strong man of the 1880's, Eugen Sandow, even in his time, proclaimed the truth that physical exercise performed mechanically and without concentration of thought could do little for the development of the muscles. He and Prof. Anderson were the first who heard of the miraculous effect of the Indian system of doing gymnastics

171

before the mirror. Unfortunately they only thought of this in connection with their exercises and thus this knowledge was soon forgotten.

It is not necessary to discuss at length the fact that Yoga philosophy is in sharp contrast to the ideas of materialism which —unfortunately—are predominant in the world today. According to Jnana Yoga, the human being consists of three parts: body, mind and soul. The soul is the SELF, the never disappearing, eternally shining, divine spark which is liberated in death from its earthly envelope of dust and continues its existence on a higher plane. The mind is the seat of the emotional and instinctive life, a little storage house of instincts, and the sub-conscious little Self which connects the perfect immaterial soul with the imperfect material body. In other words, the mind is the cloak of the soul, its semi-material, invisible garment, the storage battery of prana and cosmic rays, in contrast to our miraculously complicated, thoroughly material, precision radio transmitter and receiver, the brain. This wonder instrument receives the animating love vibrations of the GREAT TRANSMITTER and, within its smaller range, enables us to contact and exchange thoughts with other human minds. According to Yoga, animals, plants and minerals have only a mind, because in the upward line of their development they have not yet reached the stage where the divine spark within them is illuminated to give them, after thousands or millions of years, a conscious human existence.

In this connection I must contradict the mistaken notion widely held in the Occident concerning the Indian belief of 'transmigration of the soul' according to which we are reborn in animal bodies. This idea was never taught by the higher Indian religions. According to Hinduism the human soul can only be perfected in an upward direction, and there is no earthly sin which, contrary to the eternal laws of development, could cause the soul to be degraded to a lower plane of existence. On the other hand, it is an important principle of Yoga philosophy that, in order to perfect the human soul and to atone for old sins, the human being must be reborn centuries later, according to the will of God. According to the Indian view, only reincarnation can explain to any reasonable extent the—to normal human

172

standards—incomprehensible differences between people in this earthly existence. What causes one person to be born a beggar, another to be born a king, another a maharajah surrounded with treasure and crowds of attendants, and yet another as an untouchable outcast? 'Where is the justice here?' asks the Indian thinker.

Human life is a great arena in which everyone can play his own part and develop his own mental and physical faculties in a positive or negative direction according to his own free will. Has anyone ever seen a football field on which a well-fed, well-trained team would be pitted against a group of lame, weakly beggars dragged in off the street? Surely the beggars would not have a chance!

If we refuse to accept the principle of reincarnation, any kind of earthly sports arena must appear to be a most terrible injustice. According to the views generally held in the Occident by those who believe in a soul and a world to come, people are not born with mental handicaps, as their soul at birth is like a 'fresh, unwritten page'. Man receives his unspoilt, sinless soul as a gift. Yoga philosophy, however, teaches that this would be a great injustice! According to the Indian view, the inequalities of life and their meaning can only be explained when we suppose that along the upward line of mental and moral development— the final goal of which is lost in the flaming light of eternal brilliance and eternal love—there are several steps and several classes which we must repeat if we have not been successful in them before.

In our own blood-drenched times, it is impossible for a thinking person to overlook the fact that his own personal fate, the struggles of the peoples of the world, the instinctive desire for freedom and better living, and all the wars of the nations are included in a divine plan for the world. The age of materialism is coming to a close. Man is striving toward higher ideals, for he feels in his unconscious and conscious SELF that the many lies, the clash of the classes, suppression, the senseless rules of convention, and the unnatural way of living to which he is forced by a self-destroying civilization—all are in a state of decadence and collapse, and that a new, more beautiful, freer, and more open-minded, and more generous world will soon be born.

The entire system of Hatha Yoga is based on returning to a natural way of living, an intuition which guides the human mind from a higher plane. It is based on a return to an inspiration of the mind and thus becomes a valuable asset for the new world now being born and for the new generation which will lead a happier, more natural life. As the clamour of weapons dies away, a new, freer world will be born, and the time is fast approaching when we shall have to bind and heal man's wounds and train his body in a healthier, and more conscious manner. May God grant that the three greatest gifts of Hatha Yoga—health, strength, and youthfulness—may be transmitted to this new generation.

XVII

— — — — —

Helpful Hints for Yoga Pupils

GET up at the same time every morning, and go to bed at the same time every evening. Go to bed by ten o'clock at the latest; for the cosmic position of the earth *before midnight offers the nervous system the most favourable radiation for regeneration.*

Let your first thought on awakening be HEALTH! Concentrate on what health and strength mean for mind and body.

If possible, take a bath daily; free your skin of its impurities and poisons. Let your physical and mental atmosphere be pure.

As often as possible, liberate your feet from the unventilated prison of shoes; walk barefoot over the ground of forest, meadow, river bank, or lake shore. Through the soles of your feet you absorb terrestrial radiations which strengthen and refresh your organism in an extraordinary manner. City-dwellers tire so easily because shoes, concrete, and asphalt separate them from this wholesome source of energy. Out in the country, people can walk many miles without fatigue. Oft-times they take off their shoes and carry them over their shoulders! Before going to bed, exercise your toes. Move them individually so that they become animated and conscious. Practise picking up twigs and pebbles with them.

Spend a few minutes completely naked every day. You need this air bath as your skin is shut off from the air all day long and skin breathing is impeded by heavy clothing. If you begin this air bathing in the summer time and do it daily, you will soon develop a splendid resistance.

In the morning and evening do some eye exercises so that you will never be dependent on glasses.

Remember to keep your nostrils clean, as they are the

175

gateway for prana. In the morning take a nose bath by snuffing in a little moderately cool, mildly salted water. If you have catarrh, take a nose bath three times daily. Pour a little warm water, as warm as you can stand, in a dish. Stir in a level teaspoon of sodium bicarbonate, immerse your face and breathe the water into your nose until it reaches the upper cavities of your mouth; then expel and follow by practising Sarvangasana. In this way you can get rid of even the most stubborn cold.

Before and after every meal, your mouth should be rinsed out. Keep your teeth clean. Cut yourself a little twig of oak, fir or eucalyptus. The tannin freshens and strengthens your gums, preventing the formation of tartar and recession of the gums, this disease that is so common in the West. Between the bristles of your toothbrush are millions of microbes. The tannin in an oak twig acts as a disinfectant. Its use is extremely simple. Take a twig about a quarter inch in diameter and chew the end until the fibres spread out like a little brush. With this brush, clean your teeth inside and outside in a vertical direction so that both the teeth and the intervening spaces are cleaned. The crowns of your teeth have already been cleaned by your chewing the twig. Be careful not to irritate or damage your gums; instead, chew the wood until it is tender. The fresh twig is elastic, full of sap, and not so stiff as to prick your gums. Do this every second day. On the other days take a little damp salt on your index finger and when it has dissolved, rub your teeth and gums with your finger. This will increase the blood circulation. This procedure strengthens the gums and the roots of your teeth. Your teeth will be milky white and your breath fresh.

Food should be well chewed. Thorough chewing is not only necessary for digestion, but also provides an abundant flow of blood to the roots of the teeth.

Let your dietary consist more and more of raw food. If you have been a heavy meat eater, do not shift without a transitional period, as this would be harmful to the organism. The transition should be made by easy stages. A certain amount of meat eating is justified in cooler climates and is no hindrance for Yoga.

Above all be moderate! Meat causes too many wastes and toxins and places a great burden on the organs of digestion.

176

Vegetables, fruit, grains, honey, and milk products should be your chief nourishment.

See that you have a regular bowel movement daily. If your intestinal activity is not regular, the appropriate asana should be practised: Uddiyana-Bandha, Paschimotana, Yoga-Mudra, Nauli, etc. Accustom your bowels to regular movements at the natural times for elimination in the morning and after meals.

If you wish to achieve serious results in Hatha Yoga you should avoid tobacco, alcoholic drinks, and the evil habits of other dangerous vices, as all these vices deaden the very nerve centres which Yoga aims to animate.

Never allow a grudge, hate, contempt, greed, jealousy, or other base instinct to touch your mind. Such emotions set up dangerous currents, poison mind and body, and the result is sickness. Discipline your emotions; be happy and do not allow external circumstances to influence you! Always be conscious of the fact that *in the sky of your mind you are the sun*!

Speak only when you have something to say. Through unnecessary babbling, one can dissipate a tremendous amount of positive energy. Avoid wrong thinking, wrong speaking, wrong acting.

It is of great value to spend one day each month, preferably at new or full moon, in complete fasting and complete silence (Maunam). The sluice gates you close in this way enable you to accumulate energy and your will power and health to be strengthened.

If possible, practise Yoga in a special room. This room should always have pure air. Do not practise Yoga in a room filled with tobacco smoke or alcoholic smells where cheap conversations have recently been carried on! When you enter the room to practise leave outside, with your coat, all your troubles, anxiety, reluctance, and worries. Then your home will radiate happiness and consecrated purity. Practise Yoga on a clean rug or on a mat, facing east.

Begin your exercises by eliminating all feelings of fear, look to the future full of confidence, and begin the deep inhalations with faith in the healing power of the exercises. Let your soul be full of rest, gladness, patience, and determination!

177

Keep your eyes constantly on mental liberation. Strive unceasingly to attain it. Learn by heart a few sentences from the teachings of the great masters. If you feel that darkness is attacking you, drive it away with the aid of the light of the words of the masters. Where not otherwise noted, these quotations are from Swami Vivekananda.

There are two things that must be avoided:
wrong desires and mortification of the body.

Buddha

Pleasure is brief as the lightning flash—
Why then should I covet pleasures?

Buddha

The infinite future is before you, and you must always remember that each word, thought and deed, lays up a store for you and that as the bad thoughts and bad works are ready to spring upon you like tigers, so also there is the inspiring hope that the good thoughts, and good deeds, are ready with the power of a hundred thousand angels to defend you always and forever.

I must manifest the highest.
I cannot be satisfied with less.

The great motto is 'Help and not Fight', 'Assimilation and not Destruction', 'Harmony and Peace and not Dissension'.

The body is made by the thought that lies behind it.

In the strength of the individuals lies the strength of the whole nation.

It is a man-making religion that we want. We want MEN! MEN with muscles of iron and nerves of steel!

What can I do to mitigate the sufferings of my fellow men? Love them!

The powers of the mind are like rays of light dissipated; when they are concentrated they illumine. This is our only means of knowledge.

Arise! awake! and stop not till the goal is reached!

Everybody can show what evil is, but he is a friend of mankind who finds a way out of difficulty.

Man never progresses from error to truth, but from truth to truth, from lesser truth to higher truth.

If there is sin, this is the only sin—to say that you are weak, or others are weak.

This is the only way to reach the goal, to tell ourselves, and to tell everybody else, that we are divine. And as we go on repeating this, strength comes. He who falters at first will get stronger and stronger, and the voice will increase in volume until the truth takes possession of our hearts, courses through our veins, and permeates our bodies. Delusion will vanish as the light becomes more and more effulgent, load after load of ignorance will vanish, and there will come a time when all else has disappeared and the Sun alone shines.

Evil is the iron chain, good the golden one; both are chains. Be free, and know once for all that there is no chain for you. Lay hold of the golden chain to loosen the hold of the iron one, then throw both away!

Ye divinities on earth! Sinners? It is a sin to call a man so; it is a standing libel on human nature. Come up, O lions, and shake off the delusion that you are sheep, you are souls immortal, spirits free, blest and eternal; ye are not matter, ye are not bodies; matter is your servant, not you the servant of matter!

The more circumstances are against you, the more manifest becomes your inner power.

Truth is infinitely more weighty than untruth, so is goodness. If you possess these, they will make their way by sheer gravity.

Strength must come to a nation through education.

There is no want, there is no misery that you cannot remove by the consciousness of the power of the spirit within. Believe in these words and you will be omnipotent.

In a conflict between the heart and the brain, follow the heart.

To succeed, you must have tremendous perseverance, tremendous will. 'I will drink the ocean,' says the persevering soul, 'at my will mountains will crumble'. Have that sort of energy, that sort of will, work hard, and you will reach the goal.

Those who really want to be Yogis must give up, once for all, this nibbling at things. Take up one idea. Make that one idea your life; think of it; dream of it; live on that idea. Let the brain, muscles, nerves, every part of your body, be full of that idea, and just leave every other idea alone. This is the way to success, and this is the way great spiritual giants are produced.

How has all the knowledge in the world been gained but by the concentration of the powers of the mind? The world is ready to give up its secrets if we only know how to knock, how to give it the necessary blow. The strength and force of the blow come through concentration. There is no limit to the power of the human mind. The more concentrated it is, the more power is brought to bear on one point; that is the secret.

If matter is mighty, thought is almighty!

Perfection is not to be attained, it is already within us. Immortality and bliss are not to be acquired, we possess them already; they have been ours all the time. If you say you are bound, bound you will remain. If you dare declare that you are free, free you are this moment.

The salvation of the world is a cultured humanity.
Pestalozzi

If we see that which is really beautiful, we respond to it and we ourselves become a part of it. If the individual life is inspired by beauty, then the national life will accordingly CHANGE BECAUSE THE NATION DEPENDS UPON THE INDIVIDUAL.
Rukmini Devi

The SELF is not only the easiest thing to know but beyond it there is nothing else to know. All that is required to realize the SELF is to BE STILL. And what can be easier than that?
Sri Ramana Maharishi

Bring all light into the world. Light, bring light! Let light come unto everyone; the task will not be finished till everyone has reached the Lord. Bring light to the poor. Bring light to the rich, for they require it more than the poor. Bring light to the ignorant, and more light to the educated, for the vanities of the education of our time are tremendous! Thus bring light to all.

XVIII

— — — — —

Table of Practical Exercises

The aim of Hatha Yoga is to make our body conscious and to animate it! But this is not all. The final goal is also to be conscious in our understanding, that is, in our mind. Practising the asanas, together with pranayama, brings our body completely under our control. Simultaneously, however, we must remember to discipline our mind: Amidst our surroundings let us be passive and withdrawn, while at the same time we are concentrating on the SELF within us and experiencing a higher awareness. Man must keep his mind under his constant control and not allow his thoughts to drift about aimlessly; on the contrary, he must live in constant peace and equilibrium. If our thoughts acquire power over us, we no longer stand on solid ground and leave ourselves defenceless against every misfortune. The secret of happiness depends on the degree to which *we dominate our mind and our body.*

Hatha Yoga exercises teach us absolute control over the body and the energy dwelling within it. Among the exercises contained in the following tables, we find the ninth in each list is always followed by Savasana. This ninth exercise is intended to help us discipline our thoughts. When we are awake, the seat of consciousness is in the brain. Now we must force it to withdraw for a few minutes and leave our organs of thought completely empty. Our mental centre normally rests only during sleep when mother nature enables this extremely important energy reservoir to be liberated from its usual tasks.

We sit in the Padmasana posture, 'turn off' our thoughts, concentrate on our heart, and regulate our breathing until it is slow and regular. Our spine is held straight, and we experience

182

perfect peace. We focus our attention on our heart and feel as if we were 'going into' it. Leaving our troubles at the threshold, we radiate perfect quiet and peace. . . . Let us take care that no other thought disturbs us. We should practise this daily five to ten minutes! This is particularly useful and necessary for people in the Occident with an excessively active way of living.

With peace in our hearts, we lie on our back and always conclude our exercises with Savasana.

Those who practise Hatha Yoga should adapt their exercises to the goals which they wish to achieve.

For very busy office workers who practise Yoga to preserve their health, it is advisable to perform the following exercises every evening before supper—never with a full stomach!

Those who wish to develop a beautiful body and to devote more time to unfolding their consciousness should practise slow motion exercises in the morning and Yoga exercises in the evening or vice versa.

Those who wish to practise Yoga more intensively will do best to seek out a competent spiritual teacher and practise under his directions.

1ST WEEK

1. Full Yogi breathing in Padmasana or Sidhasana (pp. 116, 128/9) .. .. .. 7 x
2. Kumbhaka, 10-20 seconds retention (p. 119) 2 x
3. Ujjayi 'Sss' (p. 120) .. .. 3 x
4. Vakrasana, 1st Phase (p. 132) .. .. 2 x
5. Yoga-Mudra (p. 129) .. .. .. 3 x
6. Matsyasana (p. 132) .. .. 2 x
7. Bhujangasana (p. 137) .. .. .. 3 x
8. Viparita-Karani (p. 145) .. .. .. 3 x
9. Meditation (p. 128) .. .. 5 min.
10. Savasana (p. 154) .. .. 5 min.

2ND WEEK

1. Full Yogi Breathing, Seated (pp. 116, 128/9) 7 x
2. Kapalabhati 3 (p. 120) .. .. .. 3 x
3. Bhastrika (p. 122) .. .. 3 x
4. Sukh Purvak (p. 121) .. .. 3 x

183

5. Paschimotana (p. 133)	3 x
6. Supta-Vajrasana (p. 130)	3 x
7. Trikonasana (p. 136)	3 x
8. Sarvangasana (p. 141)	3 x
9. Meditation (p. 128)	5 min.
10. Savasana (p. 154)	5 min.

3RD WEEK

1. Full Yogi Breathing, Seated (pp. 116, 128/9)	7 x
2. Cleansing Breathing (p. 123)	3 x
3. Nerve Strengthening Breathing (p. 123) ..	3 x
4. Vakrasana 2nd Phase (p. 132)	2 x
5. Uddiyana-Bandha, Standing (p. 134) ..	3 x
6. Padahastasana (p. 134)	3 x
7. Ardha-Salabhasana (p. 139)	2 x
8. Halasana (p. 150)	2 x
9. Meditation (p. 128)	5 min.
10. Savasana (p. 154)	5 min.

4TH WEEK

1. Full Yogi Breathing, Seated (pp. 116, 128/9)	7 x
2. 'Ha' Breathing, Standing (p. 124)	2 x
3. 'Ha' Breathing, Lying (p. 124)	3 x
4. Sukh Purvak (p. 121)	3 x
5. Ardha-Bhujangasana, 1st Phase (p. 138) ..	3 x
6. Yoga-Mudra (p. 129)	3 x
7. Trikonasana (p. 136)	3 x
8. Viparita-Karani (p. 145)	3 x
9. Meditation (p. 128)	10 min.
10. Savasana (p. 154)	10 min.

5TH WEEK

1. Full Yogi Breathing, Seated (pp. 116, 128/9)	7 x
2. Pranayama No. 1 (p. 125)	3 x
3. Pranayama No. 2 (p. 125)	3 x
4. Ardha-Matsyendrasana, 2nd Phase (p. 131)	2 x
5. Paschimotana (p. 133)	3 x
6. Bhujangasana (p. 137)	3 x
7. Uddiyana-Bandha, Standing (p. 134) ..	3 x

8.	Sarvangasana (p. 141)	..	..	..	3 x
9.	Meditation (p. 128)	..	..	..	10 min.
10.	Savasana (p. 154)	..	..	..	10 min.

6TH WEEK

1.	Full Yogi Breathing, Lying (p. 116)	..	7 x
2.	Pranayama No. 3 (p. 125)	.. .. ..	2 x
3.	Pranayama No. 4 (p. 125)	.. .. ..	2 x
4.	Sukh Purvak (p. 121)	.. .. ..	3 x
5.	Yoga-Mudra (p. 129)	.. .. ..	3 x
6.	Mayurasana (p. 141)	.. .. ..	2 x
7.	Dhanurasana (p. 140)	.. .. ..	2 x
8.	Halasana (p. 150)	.. .. ..	3 x
9.	Meditation (p. 128)	.. .. ..	10 min.
10.	Savasana (p. 154)	.. .. ..	10 min.

7TH WEEK

1.	Full Yogi Breathing, Seated (pp. 116, 128/9)	7 x
2.	Pranayama No. 5 (p. 126)	3 x
3.	Pranayama No. 6 (p. 126)	3 x
4.	Ardha-Matsyendrasana, 1st Phase (p. 131)	3 x
5.	Matsyasana (p. 132)	3 x
6.	Mayurasana (p. 141)	3 x
7.	Uddiyana-Bandha, Seated (p. 134)	3 x
8.	Viparita-Karani (p. 145)	3 x
9.	Meditation (p. 128)	10 min.
10.	Savasana (p. 154)	10 min.

8TH WEEK

1.	Full Yogi Breathing, Seated (pp. 116, 128/9)	7 x
2.	Pranayama No. 7 (p. 126)	3 x
3.	Nerve Strengthening Breathing (p. 123)	2 x
4.	Sukh Purvak (p. 121)	3 x
5.	Nauli or Trikonasana (pp. 135/6)	3 x
6.	Salabhasana (p. 139)	2 x
7.	Sirshasana (p. 146)	3 x
8.	Viparita-Karani (p. 145)	3 x
9.	Meditation (p. 128)	10 min.
10.	Savasana (p. 154)	10 min.

9TH WEEK

1. Full Yogi Breathing, Seated (pp. 116, 128/9)   7 x
2. Kapalabhati (p. 120) ..   ..   3 x
3. Kumbhaka, 10-20 seconds retention (p. 119)   2 x
4. Bhastrika (p. 122)   ..   ..   3 x
5. Yoga-Mudra (p. 129)   ..   ..   ..   3 x
6. Bhujangasana (p. 137)   ..   ..   ..   2 x
7. Mayurasana (p. 141) ..   ..   3 x
8. Sirshasana (p. 146)   ..   ..   ..   3 x
9. Meditation (p. 128) ..   ..   10 min.
10. Savasana (p. 154)   ..   ..   10 min.

10TH WEEK

1. Full Yogi Breathing, Seated (pp. 116, 128/9)   7 x
2. Bhastrika (p. 122)   ..   ..   3 x
3. 'Ha' Breathing, Standing (p. 124) ..   ..   3 x
4. Simhasana, Seated (p. 153) ..   ..   ..   3 x
5. Paschimotana (p. 133)   ..   ..   ..   2 x
6. Ardha-Bhujangasana (p. 138)   ..   ..   2 x
7. Ardha-Matsyendrasana, 2nd Phase (p. 131)   2 x
8. Sarvangasana (p. 141)   ..   ..   ..   3 x
9. Meditation (p. 128) ..   ..   10 min.
10. Savasana (p. 154)   ..   ..   10 min.

11TH WEEK

1. Full Yogi Breathing, Seated (pp. 116, 128/9)   7 x
2. Ujjayi (p. 120)   ..   ..   3 x
3. 'Ha' Breathing, Lying (p. 124)   ..   ..   3 x
4. Simhasana (p. 153) ..   ..   3 x
5. Ardha-Salabhasana (p. 139) ..   ..   ..   3 x
6. Uddiyana or Nauli, Standing (pp. 134/5) ..   3 x
7. Dhanurasana (p. 140)   ..   ..   ..   2 x
8. Halasana (p. 150)   ..   ..   3 x
9. Meditation (p. 128) ..   ..   10 min.
10. Savasana (p. 154)   ..   ..   10 min.

12TH WEEK

1. Full Yogi Breathing, Seated (pp. 116, 128/9)   7 x
2. Pranayama No. 2 (p. 125) ..   ..   ..   3 x

3. Pranayama No. 7 (p. 126) .. .. .. 3 x
4. Bhastrika (p. 122) .. .. 3 x
5. Supta-Vajrasana (p. 130) .. .. .. 3 x
6. Salabhasana (p. 139) .. .. .. 3 x
7. Nauli or Uddiyana (pp. 134/5) .. .. 3 x
8. Sirshasana (p. 146) .. .. 3 x
9. Meditation (p. 128) .. .. 10 min.
10. Savasana (p. 154) .. .. 10 min.

13TH WEEK

1. Full Yogi Breathing, Seated (pp. 116, 128/9) 7 x
2. Kumbhaka, 10-20 seconds retention (p. 119) 3 x
3. Kapalabhati (p. 120) .. .. .. 3 x
4. Pranayama No. 6 (p. 126) .. .. .. 3 x
5. Yoga-Mudra (p. 129) .. .. .. 3 x
6. Ardha-Bhujangasana, 2nd Phase (p. 138) .. 3 x
7. Matsyasana (p. 132) .. .. 3 x
8. Viparita-Karani (p. 145) .. .. .. 3 x
9. Meditation (p. 128) .. .. 10 min.
10. Savasana (p. 154) .. .. 10 min.

14TH WEEK

1. Full Yogi Breathing, Seated (pp. 116, 128/9) 7 x
2. Bhastrika (p. 122) .. .. 3 x
3. Pranayama No. 4 (p. 125) .. .. .. 2 x
4. Ardha-Matsyendrasana, 2nd Phase (p. 131) 2 x
5. Trikonasana (p. 136) .. .. .. 3 x
6. Padahastasana (p. 134) .. .. .. 3 x
7. Mayurasana (p. 141) .. .. .. 3 x
8. Halasana (p. 150) .. .. 3 x
9. Meditation (p. 128) .. .. 10 min.
10. Savasana (p. 154) .. .. 10 min.

15TH WEEK

1. Full Yogi Breathing, Seated (pp. 116, 128/9) 7 x
2. 'Ha' Breathing, Lying (p. 124) .. .. 3 x
3. Pranayama No. 1 (p. 125) .. .. .. 3 x
4. Yoga-Mudra (p. 129) .. .. .. 3 x
5. Vakrasana, 2nd Phase (p. 132) .. .. 3 x

6. Ardha-Salabhasana (p. 139) .. .. .. 3 x
7. Bhujangasana (p. 137) .. .. .. 4 x
8. Sirshasana (p. 146) .. .. 3 x
9. Meditation (p. 128) .. .. 10 min.
10. Savasana (p. 154) .. .. 10 min.

16TH WEEK
1. Full Yogi Breathing, Seated (pp. 116, 128/9) 7 x
2. Nerve Strengthening Breathing (p. 123) .. 3 x
3. Pranayama No. 3 (p. 125) .. .. .. 2 x
4. Simhasana (p. 153) .. .. 3 x
5. Sirshasana (p. 146) .. .. 3 x
6. Uddiyana, Seated (p. 134) .. .. .. 3 x
7. Dhanurasana (p. 140).. .. .. .. 2 x
8. Sarvangasana (p. 141) .. .. .. 3 x
9. Meditation (p. 128) .. .. 10 min.
10. Savasana (p. 154) .. .. 10 min.

17TH WEEK
1. Full Yogi Breathing, Seated (pp. 116, 128/9) 7 x
2. Kapalabhati (p. 120) .. .. 3 x
3. Pranayama No. 7 (p. 126) .. .. .. 3 x
4. Bhastrika (p. 122) .. .. 2 x
5. Mayurasana (p. 141) .. .. 2 x
6. Dhanurasana (p. 140).. .. .. .. 2 x
7. Uddiyana, Standing (p. 134) .. .. 3 x
8. Viparita-Karani (p. 145) .. .. .. 3 x
9. Meditation (p. 128) .. .. 10 min.
10. Savasana (p. 154) .. .. 10 min.

18TH WEEK
1. Full Yogi Breathing, Seated (pp. 116, 128/9) 7 x
2. Kumbhaka, 20-30 seconds retention (p. 119) 2 x
3. Bhastrika (p. 122) .. .. 3 x
4. Sukh Purvak (p. 121) .. .. .. 2 x
5. Ardha-Matsyendrasana, 1st Phase (p. 131) 2 x
6. Trikonasana (p. 136) .. .. .. 3 x
7. Paschimotana (p. 133) .. .. .. 3 x
8. Halasana (p. 150) .. .. 3 x

9.	Meditation (p. 128)	10 min.
10.	Savasana (p. 154)	10 min.

19TH WEEK

1.	Full Yogi Breathing, Seated (pp. 116, 128/9)	7 x
2.	Ujjayi (p. 120)	5 x
3.	Pranayama No. 5. (p. 126)	3 x
4.	Sukh Purvak (p. 121)	3 x
5.	Padahastasana (p. 134)	3 x
6.	Ardha-Matsyendrasana, 2nd Phase (p. 131)	3 x
7.	Uddiyana-Bandha, Standing (p. 134) ..	3 x
8.	Sarvangasana (p. 141)	3 x
9.	Meditation (p. 128)	10 min.
10.	Savasana (p. 154)	10 min.

20TH WEEK

1.	Full Yogi Breathing, Seated (pp. 116, 128/9)	7 x
2.	'Ha' Breathing, Lying (p. 124)	3 x
3.	Pranayama No. 4 (p. 125)	3 x
4.	Sirshasana (p. 146)	3 x
5.	Supta-Vajrasana (p. 130)	2 x
6.	Uddiyana-Bandha, Seated (p. 134)	3 x
7.	Dhanurasana (p. 140)..	2 x
8.	Viparita-Karani (p. 145)	3 x
9.	Meditation (p. 128)	10 min.
10.	Savasana (p. 154)	10 min.

21ST WEEK

1.	Full Yogi Breathing, Seated (pp. 116, 128/9)	7 x
2.	Bhastrika (p. 122)	3 x
3.	Kumbhaka, 20-30 seconds retention (p. 119)	3 x
4.	Pranayama No. 4 (p. 125)	2 x
5.	Yoga-Mudra (p. 129)	3 x
6.	Mayurasana (p. 141)	3 x
7.	Ardha-Matsyendrasana, 2nd Phase (p. 131)	2 x
8.	Sirshasana (p. 146)	3 x
9.	Meditation (p. 128)	10 min.
10.	Savasana (p. 154)	10 min.

189

As may be seen from the above tables, each series of exercises lasts a total of approximately twenty-five to forty minutes. After completing the series, everyone is free to practise the pranayama and asanas that he has already learnt and which appeal to him. It is not recommended, however, to practise more than an hour at a time.

* * *

I warmly commend both pranayama and the asanas as well as the ancient system of physical exercises which combine belief, will power, and imagination, to the physical training teachers of the Occident. It is very much worth while to devote one's careful attention to this venerable science, and it would be very useful to give children in their earliest years the benefit of Hatha Yoga. This would develop a new generation with new strength, self discipline, and strong will power; for *only when the body is healthy is it an adaptable and obedient instrument for manifesting the* SELF.